DAT Quantitative Reasoning Exercise Book

www.EffortlessMath.com

... So Much More Online!

✓ FREE Math lessons

✓ More Math learning books!

✓ Mathematics Worksheets

✓ Online Math Tutors

Need a PDF version of this book?

Please visit www.EffortlessMath.com

DAT Quantitative Reasoning Exercise Book

Student Workbook and Two Realistic

DAT Quantitative Reasoning Tests

By

Reza Nazari & Ava Ross

Copyright © 2019

Reza Nazari & Ava Ross

All rights reserved. No part of this publication may be reproduced, stored in a retrieval system, or transmitted in any form or by any means, electronic, mechanical, photocopying, recording, scanning, or otherwise, except as permitted under Section 107 or 108 of the 1976 United States Copyright Ac, without permission of the author.

All inquiries should be addressed to:

info@effortlessMath.com

www.EffortlessMath.com

ISBN-13: 978-1-970036-78-7

ISBN-10: 1-970036-78-8

Published by: Effortless Math Education

www.EffortlessMath.com

Description

Get ready for the DAT Quantitative Reasoning Test with a PERFECT Workbook!

DAT Quantitative Reasoning Exercise book, which reflects the 2019 test guidelines and topics, is dedicated to preparing test takers to ace the DAT Quantitative Reasoning Test. This DAT workbook's new edition has been updated to replicate questions appearing on the most recent DAT tests. Here is intensive preparation for the DAT Quantitative Reasoning test, and a precious learning tool for test takers who need extra practice in Math to raise their DAT scores. After completing this workbook, you will have solid foundation and adequate practice that is necessary to ace the DAT Quantitative Reasoning test. **This workbook is your ticket to score higher on DAT Quantitative Reasoning.**

The updated version of this hands-on workbook represents extensive exercises, quantitative reasoning problems, sample DAT questions, and quizzes with answers and detailed solutions to help you hone your quantitative reasoning skills, overcome your exam anxiety, and boost your confidence -- and do your best to defeat DAT exam on test day.

Each of Math exercises is answered in the book and we have provided explanation of the answers for the two full-length DAT Quantitative Reasoning practice tests as well which will help test takers find their weak areas and raise their scores. This is a unique and perfect practice book to beat the DAT Test.

Separate Math chapters offer a complete review of the DAT Quantitative Reasoning test, including:

- ✓ Arithmetic and Number Operations
- ✓ Algebra and Functions,
- ✓ Geometry and Measurement
- ✓ Data analysis, Statistics, & Probability
- ✓ … and also includes **two full-length practice tests!**

The surest way to succeed on DAT Quantitative Reasoning Test is with intensive practice in every Math topic tested--and that's what you will get in ***DAT Quantitative Reasoning Exercise Book***. Each chapter of this focused format has a comprehensive review created by Test Prep experts that goes into detail to cover all of the content likely to appear on the DAT test. Not only does this all-inclusive workbook offer everything you will ever need to conquer DAT Quantitative

Reasoning test, it also contains two full-length and realistic DAT Quantitative Reasoning tests that reflect the format and question types on the DAT to help you check your exam-readiness and identify where you need more practice.

Effortless Quantitative Reasoning Workbook *for the DAT Test* contains many exciting and unique features to help you improve your test scores, including:

- ✓ Content 100% aligned with the 2019 DAT test
- ✓ Written by DAT Quantitative Reasoning tutors and test experts
- ✓ Complete coverage of all DAT Math concepts and topics which you will be tested
- ✓ Over 2,500 additional DAT Math practice questions in both multiple-choice and grid-in formats with answers grouped by topic, so you can focus on your weak areas
- ✓ Abundant Math skill building exercises to help test-takers approach different question types that might be unfamiliar to them
- ✓ Exercises on different DAT Math topics such as integers, percent, equations, polynomials, exponents and radicals
- ✓ 2 full-length practice tests (featuring new question types) with detailed answers

This DAT Quantitative Reasoning Workbook and other Effortless Quantitative Reasoning Education books are used by thousands of students each year to help them review core content areas, brush-up in Math, discover their strengths and weaknesses, and achieve their best scores on the DAT test.

Do NOT take the DAT test without reviewing the Math questions in this workbook!

About the Author

Reza Nazari is the author of more than 100 Math learning books including:
– **Math and Critical Thinking Challenges:** For the Middle and High School Student
– **DAT Quantitative Reasoning in 30 Days**
– **ASVAB Math Workbook 2018 - 2019**
– **Effortless Math Education Workbooks**
– **and many more mathematics books ...**

Reza is also an experienced Math instructor and a test–prep expert who has been tutoring students since 2008. Reza is the founder of Effortless Math Education, a tutoring company that has helped many students raise their standardized test scores—and attend the colleges of their dreams. Reza provides an individualized custom learning plan and the personalized attention that makes a difference in how students view Math.

You can contact Reza via email at:
reza@EffortlessMath.com

Find Reza's professional profile at:
goo.gl/zoC9rJ

Contents

Chapter 1: Fundamental and Building Blocks 10

    Simplifying Fractions 11

    Adding and Subtracting Fractions 12

    Multiplying and Dividing Fractions 13

    Adding and Subtracting Mixed Numbers 14

    Multiplying and Dividing Mixed Numbers 15

    Adding and Subtracting Decimals 16

    Multiplying and Dividing Decimals 17

    Comparing Decimals 18

    Rounding Decimals 19

    Factoring Numbers 20

    Greatest Common Factor 21

    Least Common Multiple 22

    Answers of Worksheets – Chapter 1 23

Chapter 2: Real Numbers and Integers 27

    Adding and Subtracting Integers 28

    Multiplying and Dividing Integers 29

    Order of Operations 30

    Ordering Integers and Numbers 31

    Integers and Absolute Value 32

    Answers of Worksheets – Chapter 2 33

Chapter 3: Proportions, Ratios, and Percent 35

    Simplifying Ratios 36

    Proportional Ratios 37

    Similarity and Ratios 38

    Ratio and Rates Word Problems 39

    Percentage Calculations 40

    Percent Problems 41

    Discount, Tax and Tip 42

    Percent of Change 43

Simple Interest 44

Answers of Worksheets – Chapter 3 45

Chapter 4: Algebraic Expressions 48

Simplifying Variable Expressions 49

Simplifying Polynomial Expressions 50

Translate Phrases into an Algebraic Statement 51

The Distributive Property 52

Evaluating One Variable Expressions 53

Evaluating Two Variables Expressions 54

Combining like Terms 55

Answers of Worksheets – Chapter 4 56

Chapter 5: Equations and Inequalities 58

One–Step Equations 59

Multi–Step Equations 60

Graphing Single–Variable Inequalities 61

One–Step Inequalities 62

Multi-Step Inequalities 63

Systems of Equations 64

Systems of Equations Word Problems 65

Quadratic Equation 66

Answers of Worksheets – Chapter 5 67

Chapter 6: Linear Functions 70

Finding Slope 71

Graphing Lines Using Line Equation 72

Writing Linear Equations 73

Graphing Linear Inequalities 74

Finding Midpoint 75

Finding Distance of Two Points 76

Answers of Worksheets – Chapter 6 77

Chapter 7: Exponents 80

Multiplication Property of Exponents 81

Zero and Negative Exponents 82

Division Property of Exponents 83

Powers of Products and Quotients 84

Negative Exponents and Negative Bases 85

Scientific Notation 86

Answers of Worksheets – Chapter 7 87

Chapter 8: Polynomials 90

Writing Polynomials in Standard Form 91

Simplifying Polynomials 92

Adding and Subtracting Polynomials 93

Multiplying Monomials 94

Multiplying and Dividing Monomials 95

Multiplying a Polynomial and a Monomial 96

Multiplying Binomials 97

Factoring Trinomials 98

Operations with Polynomials 99

Answers of Worksheets – Chapter 8 100

Chapter 9: Functions Operations 104

Evaluating Function 105

Adding and Subtracting Functions 106

Multiplying and Dividing Functions 107

Composition of Functions 108

Answers of Worksheets – Chapter 9 109

Chapter 10: Quadratic 111

Solving Quadratic Equations 112

Quadratic Formula and the Discriminant 113

Quadratic Inequalities 114

Graphing Quadratic Functions 115

Answers of Worksheets – Chapter 10 116

Chapter 11: Radical Expressions 118

Simplifying Radical Expressions 119

Multiplying Radical Expressions 120

Simplifying Radical Expressions Involving Fractions 121

Adding and Subtracting Radical Expressions 122

Domain and Range of Radical Functions 123

Solving Radical Equations 124

Answers of Worksheets – Chapter 11 125

Chapter 12: Geometry and Solid Figures 129

Angles 130

Pythagorean Relationship 131

Triangles 132

Polygons 133

Trapezoids 134

Circles 135

Cubes 136

Rectangular Prism 137

Cylinder 138

Pyramids and Cone 139

Answers of Worksheets – Chapter 12 140

Chapter 13: Statistics and Probability 142

Mean and Median 143

Mode and Range 144

Pie Graph 145

Probability Problems 146

Factorials 147

Combinations and Permutations 148

Answers of Worksheets – Chapter 13 149

Chapter 14: Trigonometric Functions 151

Trig ratios of General Angles 152

Sketch Each Angle in Standard Position 153

Angles and Angle Measure 154

Evaluating Trigonometric Functions 155

Missing Sides and Angles of a Right Triangle 156

Arc Length and Sector Area 157

Answers of Worksheets – Chapter 14 158

DAT Test Review 161

DAT Quantitative Reasoning Practice Tests 162

DAT Quantitative Reasoning Practice Tests Answers and Explanations 196

Chapter 1:
Fundamental and Building Blocks

Topics that you'll practice in this chapter:

- ✓ Simplifying Fractions
- ✓ Adding and Subtracting Fractions
- ✓ Multiplying and Dividing Fractions
- ✓ Adding and Subtract Mixed Numbers
- ✓ Multiplying and Dividing Mixed Numbers
- ✓ Adding and Subtracting Decimals
- ✓ Multiplying and Dividing Decimals
- ✓ Comparing Decimals
- ✓ Rounding Decimals
- ✓ Factoring Numbers
- ✓ Greatest Common Factor
- ✓ Least Common Multiple

"A Man is like a fraction whose numerator is what he is and whose denominator is what he thinks of himself. The larger the denominator, the smaller the fraction." –Tolstoy

Simplifying Fractions

✎ **Simplify each fraction to its lowest terms.**

1) $\frac{9}{18} =$

2) $\frac{8}{10} =$

3) $\frac{6}{8} =$

4) $\frac{5}{20} =$

5) $\frac{18}{24} =$

6) $\frac{6}{9} =$

7) $\frac{12}{15} =$

8) $\frac{4}{16} =$

9) $\frac{18}{36} =$

10) $\frac{6}{42} =$

11) $\frac{13}{39} =$

12) $\frac{21}{28} =$

13) $\frac{63}{77} =$

14) $\frac{36}{40} =$

15) $\frac{21}{63} =$

16) $\frac{30}{84} =$

17) $\frac{50}{125} =$

18) $\frac{72}{108} =$

19) $\frac{49}{112} =$

20) $\frac{240}{320} =$

21) $\frac{120}{150} =$

✎ **Solve each problem.**

22) Which of the following fractions equal to $\frac{4}{5}$? _____

  A. $\frac{64}{75}$ B. $\frac{92}{115}$ C. $\frac{60}{85}$ D. $\frac{160}{220}$

23) Which of the following fractions equal to $\frac{3}{7}$? _____

  A. $\frac{63}{147}$ B. $\frac{75}{182}$ C. $\frac{54}{140}$ D. $\frac{39}{98}$

24) Which of the following fractions equal to $\frac{2}{9}$? _____

  A. $\frac{84}{386}$ B. $\frac{52}{234}$ C. $\frac{96}{450}$ D. $\frac{112}{522}$

Adding and Subtracting Fractions

✎ **Find the sum.**

1) $\frac{1}{3} + \frac{2}{3} =$

2) $\frac{1}{2} + \frac{1}{3} =$

3) $\frac{2}{5} + \frac{1}{2} =$

4) $\frac{3}{7} + \frac{2}{3} =$

5) $\frac{3}{4} + \frac{2}{5} =$

6) $\frac{3}{5} + \frac{1}{5} =$

7) $\frac{5}{9} + \frac{1}{2} =$

8) $\frac{3}{5} + \frac{3}{8} =$

9) $\frac{5}{9} + \frac{3}{7} =$

10) $\frac{5}{11} + \frac{1}{4} =$

11) $\frac{3}{7} + \frac{1}{6} =$

12) $\frac{3}{14} + \frac{3}{4} =$

✎ **Find the difference.**

13) $\frac{1}{2} - \frac{1}{3} =$

14) $\frac{4}{5} - \frac{2}{3} =$

15) $\frac{2}{3} - \frac{1}{6} =$

16) $\frac{3}{5} - \frac{1}{2} =$

17) $\frac{8}{9} - \frac{2}{5} =$

18) $\frac{4}{7} - \frac{1}{9} =$

19) $\frac{2}{5} - \frac{1}{4} =$

20) $\frac{5}{8} - \frac{2}{6} =$

21) $\frac{4}{15} - \frac{1}{10} =$

22) $\frac{7}{20} - \frac{1}{5} =$

23) $\frac{3}{18} - \frac{1}{12} =$

24) $\frac{9}{24} - \frac{3}{16} =$

25) $\frac{3}{7} - \frac{2}{5} =$

26) $\frac{5}{9} - \frac{1}{6} =$

27) $\frac{2}{5} - \frac{1}{10} =$

28) $\frac{5}{12} - \frac{2}{9} =$

29) $\frac{2}{13} - \frac{3}{7} =$

30) $\frac{4}{11} - \frac{5}{8} =$

Multiplying and Dividing Fractions

✎ **Find the value of each expression in lowest terms.**

1) $\frac{1}{2} \times \frac{3}{4} =$

2) $\frac{3}{5} \times \frac{2}{3} =$

3) $\frac{1}{4} \times \frac{2}{5} =$

4) $\frac{1}{6} \times \frac{4}{5} =$

5) $\frac{1}{5} \times \frac{1}{4} =$

6) $\frac{2}{5} \times \frac{1}{2} =$

7) $\frac{7}{9} \times \frac{1}{3} =$

8) $\frac{5}{7} \times \frac{3}{8} =$

9) $\frac{8}{9} \times \frac{6}{7} =$

10) $\frac{5}{6} \times \frac{3}{5} =$

11) $\frac{3}{8} \times \frac{1}{9} =$

12) $\frac{1}{12} \times \frac{3}{7} =$

✎ **Find the value of each expression in lowest terms.**

13) $\frac{1}{2} \div \frac{1}{4} =$

14) $\frac{1}{3} \div \frac{1}{2} =$

15) $\frac{2}{5} \div \frac{1}{3} =$

16) $\frac{1}{4} \div \frac{2}{3} =$

17) $\frac{1}{5} \div \frac{3}{10} =$

18) $\frac{2}{7} \div \frac{1}{3} =$

19) $\frac{3}{5} \div \frac{5}{9} =$

20) $\frac{2}{23} \div \frac{2}{9} =$

21) $\frac{4}{13} \div \frac{1}{4} =$

22) $\frac{9}{14} \div \frac{3}{7} =$

23) $\frac{8}{15} \div \frac{2}{5} =$

24) $\frac{2}{9} \div \frac{7}{11} =$

25) $\frac{2}{5} \div \frac{3}{4} =$

26) $\frac{4}{11} \div \frac{2}{5} =$

27) $\frac{2}{15} \div \frac{5}{8} =$

28) $\frac{3}{10} \div \frac{2}{5} =$

29) $\frac{4}{5} \div \frac{3}{7} =$

30) $\frac{2}{11} \div \frac{3}{5} =$

Adding and Subtracting Mixed Numbers

✎ **Find the sum.**

1) $2\frac{1}{2} + 1\frac{1}{3} =$

2) $6\frac{1}{2} + 3\frac{1}{2} =$

3) $2\frac{3}{8} + 3\frac{1}{8} =$

4) $4\frac{1}{2} + 1\frac{1}{4} =$

5) $1\frac{3}{7} + 1\frac{5}{14} =$

6) $6\frac{5}{12} + 3\frac{3}{4} =$

7) $5\frac{1}{2} + 8\frac{3}{4} =$

8) $3\frac{7}{8} + 3\frac{1}{3} =$

9) $3\frac{3}{9} + 7\frac{6}{11} =$

10) $7\frac{5}{12} + 4\frac{3}{10} =$

✎ **Find the difference.**

11) $3\frac{1}{3} - 1\frac{1}{3} =$

12) $4\frac{1}{2} - 3\frac{1}{2} =$

13) $5\frac{1}{2} - 2\frac{1}{4} =$

14) $6\frac{1}{6} - 5\frac{1}{3} =$

15) $8\frac{1}{2} - 1\frac{1}{10} =$

16) $9\frac{1}{2} - 2\frac{1}{4} =$

17) $9\frac{1}{5} - 5\frac{1}{6} =$

18) $14\frac{3}{10} - 13\frac{1}{3} =$

19) $19\frac{2}{3} - 11\frac{5}{8} =$

20) $20\frac{3}{4} - 14\frac{2}{3} =$

21) $2\frac{1}{2} - 1\frac{1}{5} =$

22) $3\frac{1}{6} - 1\frac{1}{10} =$

23) $16\frac{2}{7} - 11\frac{2}{3} =$

24) $15\frac{1}{7} - 10\frac{1}{8} =$

25) $12\frac{3}{4} - 7\frac{1}{3} =$

26) $15\frac{2}{5} - 5\frac{2}{3} =$

Multiplying and Dividing Mixed Numbers

✎ **Find the product.**

1) $4\frac{1}{3} \times 2\frac{1}{5} =$

2) $3\frac{1}{2} \times 3\frac{1}{4} =$

3) $5\frac{2}{5} \times 2\frac{1}{3} =$

4) $2\frac{1}{2} \times 1\frac{2}{9} =$

5) $3\frac{4}{7} \times 2\frac{3}{5} =$

6) $7\frac{2}{3} \times 2\frac{2}{3} =$

7) $9\frac{8}{9} \times 8\frac{3}{4} =$

8) $2\frac{4}{7} \times 5\frac{2}{9} =$

9) $5\frac{2}{5} \times 2\frac{3}{5} =$

10) $3\frac{5}{7} \times 3\frac{5}{6} =$

✎ **Find the quotient.**

11) $1\frac{2}{3} \div 3\frac{1}{3} =$

12) $2\frac{1}{4} \div 1\frac{1}{2} =$

13) $10\frac{1}{2} \div 1\frac{2}{3} =$

14) $3\frac{1}{6} \div 4\frac{2}{3} =$

15) $4\frac{1}{8} \div 2\frac{1}{2} =$

16) $2\frac{1}{10} \div 2\frac{3}{5} =$

17) $1\frac{4}{11} \div 1\frac{1}{4} =$

18) $9\frac{1}{2} \div 9\frac{2}{3} =$

19) $8\frac{3}{4} \div 2\frac{2}{5} =$

20) $12\frac{1}{2} \div 9\frac{1}{3} =$

21) $2\frac{1}{8} \div 1\frac{1}{2} =$

22) $1\frac{1}{10} \div 1\frac{3}{5} =$

23) $5\frac{2}{5} \div 1\frac{3}{4} =$

24) $5\frac{1}{2} \div 2\frac{2}{3} =$

25) $3\frac{3}{4} \div 1\frac{1}{5} =$

26) $3\frac{1}{2} \div 1\frac{1}{3} =$

Adding and Subtracting Decimals

✍ **Add and subtract decimals.**

1) 31.13
   $-\ 11.45$
   _____

4) 56.67
   $-\ 44.39$
   _____

7) 66.24
   $-\ 23.11$
   _____

2) 35.25
   $+\ 24.47$
   _____

5) 71.47
   $+\ 16.25$
   _____

8) 39.75
   $+\ 12.85$
   _____

3) 73.50
   $+\ 22.78$
   _____

6) 68.99
   $-\ 53.61$
   _____

9) 229.25
   $-\ 84.67$
   _____

✍ **Find the missing number.**

10) ___ + 2.5 = 3.9

11) 1.7 + ___ = 4.98

12) 5.25 + ___ = 7

13) 6.55 − ___ = 2.45

14) ___ − 3.98 = 5.32

15) ___ − 11.67 = 14.48

16) 12.35 + ___ = 14.78

17) ___ − 23.89 = 13.90

18) ___ + 17.28 = 19.56

19) 77.90 + ___ = 102.60

Multiplying and Dividing Decimals

✍ **Find the product.**

1) $0.5 \times 0.4 =$

2) $2.5 \times 0.2 =$

3) $1.25 \times 0.5 =$

4) $0.75 \times 0.2 =$

5) $1.92 \times 0.8 =$

6) $0.55 \times 0.4 =$

7) $3.24 \times 1.2 =$

8) $12.5 \times 4.2 =$

9) $22.6 \times 8.2 =$

10) $17.2 \times 4.5 =$

11) $25.1 \times 12.5 =$

12) $33.2 \times 2.2 =$

✍ **Find the quotient.**

13) $1.67 \div 100 =$

14) $52.2 \div 1,000 =$

15) $4.2 \div 2 =$

16) $8.6 \div 0.5 =$

17) $12.6 \div 0.2 =$

18) $16.5 \div 5 =$

19) $13.25 \div 100 =$

20) $25.6 \div 0.4 =$

21) $28.24 \div 0.1 =$

22) $34.16 \div 0.25 =$

23) $44.28 \div 0.5 =$

24) $38.78 \div 0.02 =$

Comparing Decimals

✎ **Write the correct comparison symbol (>, < or =).**

1) 0.50 ☐ 0.050

2) 0.025 ☐ 0.25

3) 2.060 ☐ 2.07

4) 1.75 ☐ 1.07

5) 4.04 ☐ 0.440

6) 3.05 ☐ 3.5

7) 5.05 ☐ 5.050

8) 1.02 ☐ 1.1

9) 2.45 ☐ 2.125

10) 0.932 ☐ 0.0932

11) 3.15 ☐ 3.150

12) 0.718 ☐ 0.89

13) 7.060 ☐ 7.60

14) 3.59 ☐ 3.129

15) 4.33 ☐ 4.319

16) 2.25 ☐ 2.250

17) 1.95 ☐ 1.095

18) 8.051 ☐ 8.50

19) 1.022 ☐ 1.020

20) 3.77 ☐ 3.770

Rounding Decimals

✎ **Round each decimal to the nearest whole number.**

1) 23.18   3) 14.45   5) 3.95

2) 8.6   4) 7.5   6) 56.7

✎ **Round each decimal to the nearest tenth.**

7) 22.652   9) 47.847   11) 16.184

8) 30.342   10) 82.88   12) 71.79

✎ **Round each decimal to the nearest hundredth.**

13) 5.439   15) 26.1855   17) 91.448

14) 12.907   16) 48.623   18) 29.354

✎ **Round each decimal to the nearest thousandth.**

19) 14.67374   21) 78.7191   23) 10.0678

20) 7.54647   22) 70.2732   24) 46.54765

Factoring Numbers

✎ *List all positive factors of each number.*

1) 8

2) 9

3) 15

4) 16

5) 25

6) 28

7) 26

8) 35

9) 42

10) 48

11) 50

12) 36

13) 55

14) 40

15) 62

16) 84

17) 75

18) 68

19) 96

20) 78

21) 94

22) 82

23) 81

24) 72

Greatest Common Factor

✎ **Find the GCF for each number pair.**

1) 4, 2

2) 3, 5

3) 2, 6

4) 4, 7

5) 5, 10

6) 6, 12

7) 7, 14

8) 6, 14

9) 5, 12

10) 4, 14

11) 15, 18

12) 12, 20

13) 12, 16

14) 15, 27

15) 8, 24

16) 28, 16

17) 32, 24

18) 18, 36

19) 26, 20

20) 30, 14

21) 24, 20

22) 14, 22

23) 25, 15

24) 28, 32

Least Common Multiple

✍ **Find the LCM for each number pair.**

1) 3, 6

2) 5, 10

3) 6, 14

4) 8, 9

5) 6, 18

6) 10, 12

7) 4, 12

8) 5, 15

9) 4, 18

10) 9, 12

11) 12, 16

12) 15, 18

13) 8, 24

14) 9, 28

15) 12, 24

16) 15, 20

17) 25, 18

18) 27, 24

19) 28, 18

20) 16, 30

21) 14, 28

22) 20, 35

23) 25, 30

24) 32, 27

Answers of Worksheets – Chapter 1

Simplifying Fractions

1) $\frac{1}{2}$
2) $\frac{4}{5}$
3) $\frac{3}{4}$
4) $\frac{1}{4}$
5) $\frac{3}{4}$
6) $\frac{2}{3}$
7) $\frac{4}{5}$
8) $\frac{1}{4}$
9) $\frac{1}{2}$
10) $\frac{1}{7}$
11) $\frac{1}{3}$
12) $\frac{3}{4}$
13) $\frac{9}{11}$
14) $\frac{9}{10}$
15) $\frac{1}{3}$
16) $\frac{5}{14}$
17) $\frac{2}{5}$
18) $\frac{2}{3}$
19) $\frac{7}{16}$
20) $\frac{3}{4}$
21) $\frac{4}{5}$
22) B
23) A
24) B

Adding and Subtracting Fractions

1) $\frac{3}{3} = 1$
2) $\frac{5}{6}$
3) $\frac{9}{10}$
4) $\frac{23}{21}$
5) $\frac{23}{20}$
6) $\frac{4}{5}$
7) $\frac{19}{18}$
8) $\frac{39}{40}$
9) $\frac{62}{63}$
10) $\frac{31}{44}$
11) $\frac{25}{42}$
12) $\frac{27}{28}$
13) $\frac{1}{6}$
14) $\frac{2}{15}$
15) $\frac{1}{2}$
16) $\frac{1}{10}$
17) $\frac{22}{45}$
18) $\frac{29}{63}$
19) $\frac{3}{20}$
20) $\frac{7}{24}$
21) $\frac{1}{6}$
22) $\frac{3}{20}$
23) $\frac{1}{12}$
24) $\frac{3}{16}$
25) $\frac{1}{35}$
26) $\frac{7}{18}$
27) $\frac{3}{10}$
28) $\frac{7}{36}$
29) $-\frac{25}{91}$
30) $-\frac{15}{88}$

Multiplying and Dividing Fractions

1) $\frac{3}{8}$
2) $\frac{2}{5}$
3) $\frac{1}{10}$
4) $\frac{2}{15}$
5) $\frac{1}{20}$
6) $\frac{1}{5}$
7) $\frac{7}{27}$
8) $\frac{15}{56}$
9) $\frac{16}{21}$

10) $\frac{1}{2}$
11) $\frac{1}{24}$
12) $\frac{1}{28}$
13) 2
14) $\frac{2}{3}$
15) $\frac{6}{5}$
16) $\frac{3}{8}$

17) $\frac{2}{3}$
18) $\frac{6}{7}$
19) $\frac{27}{25}$
20) $\frac{9}{23}$
21) $\frac{16}{13}$
22) $\frac{21}{14}$
23) $\frac{4}{3}$

24) $\frac{22}{63}$
25) $\frac{8}{15}$
26) $\frac{10}{11}$
27) $\frac{16}{75}$
28) $\frac{3}{4}$
29) $\frac{28}{15}$
30) $\frac{10}{33}$

Adding and Subtracting Mixed Numbers

1) $3\frac{5}{6}$
2) 10
3) $5\frac{1}{2}$
4) $5\frac{3}{4}$
5) $2\frac{11}{14}$
6) $10\frac{1}{6}$
7) $14\frac{1}{4}$
8) $7\frac{5}{24}$
9) $10\frac{29}{33}$

10) $11\frac{43}{60}$
11) 2
12) 1
13) $3\frac{1}{4}$
14) $\frac{5}{6}$
15) $7\frac{2}{5}$
16) $7\frac{1}{4}$
17) $4\frac{1}{30}$
18) $\frac{29}{30}$

19) $8\frac{1}{24}$
20) $6\frac{1}{12}$
21) $\frac{13}{10}$
22) $2\frac{1}{15}$
23) $4\frac{13}{21}$
24) $5\frac{1}{56}$
25) $5\frac{5}{12}$
26) $9\frac{11}{15}$

Multiplying and Dividing Mixed Numbers

1) $9\frac{8}{15}$
2) $11\frac{3}{8}$
3) $12\frac{3}{5}$
4) $3\frac{1}{18}$
5) $9\frac{2}{7}$
6) $20\frac{4}{9}$
7) $86\frac{19}{36}$
8) $13\frac{3}{7}$

9) $14\frac{1}{25}$
10) $14\frac{5}{21}$
11) $\frac{1}{2}$
12) $1\frac{1}{2}$
13) $6\frac{3}{10}$
14) $\frac{19}{28}$
15) $1\frac{13}{20}$

16) $\frac{21}{26}$
17) $1\frac{1}{11}$
18) $\frac{57}{58}$
19) $3\frac{31}{48}$
20) $1\frac{19}{56}$
21) $1\frac{5}{12}$
22) $\frac{11}{16}$

23) $3\frac{3}{35}$
24) $2\frac{1}{16}$
25) $3\frac{1}{8}$
26) $2\frac{5}{8}$

Adding and Subtracting Decimals

1) 19.68
2) 59.72
3) 96.28
4) 12.28
5) 87.72
6) 15.38
7) 43.13
8) 52.60
9) 144.58
10) 1.4
11) 3.28
12) 1.75
13) 4.1
14) 9.3
15) 26.15
16) 2.43
17) 37.79
18) 2.28
19) 24.7

Multiplying and Dividing Decimals

1) 0.2
2) 0.5
3) 0.625
4) 0.15
5) 1.536
6) 0.22
7) 3.888
8) 52.5
9) 185.32
10) 77.4
11) 313.75
12) 73.04
13) 0.0167
14) 0.0522
15) 2.1
16) 4.3
17) 63
18) 3.3
19) 0.1325
20) 64
21) 282.4
22) 136.64
23) 88.56
24) 1,939

Comparing Decimals

1) >
2) <
3) <
4) >
5) >
6) <
7) =
8) <
9) >
10) >
11) =
12) <
13) <
14) >
15) >
16) =
17) >
18) <
19) >
20) =

Rounding Decimals

1) 23
2) 9
3) 14
4) 8
5) 4
6) 57
7) 22.7
8) 30.3
9) 47.8
10) 82.9
11) 16.2
12) 71.8
13) 5.44
14) 12.91
15) 26.19
16) 48.62
17) 91.45
18) 29.35
19) 14.674
20) 7.546
21) 78.719
22) 70.273
23) 10.068
24) 46.548

Factoring Numbers

1) 1, 2, 4, 8
2) 1, 3, 9
3) 1, 3, 5, 15
4) 1, 2, 4, 8, 16
5) 1, 5, 25
6) 1, 2, 4, 7, 14, 28
7) 1, 2, 13, 26
8) 1, 5, 7, 35
9) 1, 2, 3, 6, 7, 14, 21, 42
10) 1, 2, 3, 4, 6, 8, 12, 16, 24, 48
11) 1, 2, 5, 10, 25, 50
12) 1, 2, 3, 4, 6, 9, 12, 18, 36
13) 1, 5, 11, 55
14) 1, 2, 4, 5, 8, 10, 20, 40
15) 1, 2, 31, 62
16) 1, 2, 3, 4, 6, 7, 12, 14, 21, 28, 42, 84
17) 1, 3, 5, 15, 25, 75
18) 1, 2, 4, 17, 34, 68
19) 1, 2, 3, 4, 6, 8, 12, 16, 24, 32, 48, 96
20) 1, 2, 3, 6, 13, 26, 39, 78
21) 1, 2, 47, 94
22) 1, 2, 41, 82
23) 1, 3, 9, 27, 81
24) 1, 2, 3, 4, 6, 8, 9, 12, 18, 24, 36, 72

Greatest Common Factor

1) 2
2) 1
3) 2
4) 1
5) 5
6) 6
7) 7
8) 2
9) 1
10) 2
11) 3
12) 4
13) 4
14) 3
15) 8
16) 4
17) 8
18) 18
19) 2
20) 2
21) 4
22) 2
23) 5
24) 4

Least Common Multiple

1) 6
2) 10
3) 42
4) 72
5) 18
6) 60
7) 12
8) 15
9) 36
10) 36
11) 48
12) 90
13) 24
14) 252
15) 24
16) 60
17) 450
18) 216
19) 252
20) 240
21) 28
22) 140
23) 150
24) 864

Chapter 2:

Real Numbers and Integers

Topics that you'll practice in this chapter:

✓ Adding and Subtracting Integers

✓ Multiplying and Dividing Integers

✓ Order of Operations

✓ Ordering Integers and Numbers

✓ Integers and Absolute Value

"If people do not believe that Mathematics is simple, it is only because they do not realize how complicated life is." — John von Neumann

Adding and Subtracting Integers

✍ *Find each sum.*

1) $12 + (-5) =$

2) $(-14) + (-18) =$

3) $8 + (-28) =$

4) $43 + (-12) =$

5) $(-7) + (-11) + 4 =$

6) $37 + (-16) + 12 =$

7) $29 + (-21) + (-12) + 20 =$

8) $(-15) + (-25) + 18 + 25 =$

9) $30 + (-28) + (35 - 32) =$

10) $25 + (-15) + (44 - 17) =$

✍ *Find each difference.*

11) $(-12) - (-8) =$

12) $15 - (-20) =$

13) $(-11) - 25 =$

14) $30 - (-16) =$

15) $56 - (45 - 23) =$

16) $15 - (-4) - (-34) =$

17) $(24 + 14) - (-55) =$

18) $23 - 15 - (-3) =$

19) $49 - (15 + 12) - (-4) =$

20) $29 - (-17) - (-25) =$

21) $12 - (-8) - (-18) =$

22) $(15 - 28) - (-22) =$

23) $19 - 44 - (-14) =$

24) $67 - (57 + 19) - (-8) =$

25) $56 - (-12) + (-19) =$

26) $22 - (-44) + (-55) =$

Multiplying and Dividing Integers

✎ **Find each product.**

1) $(-7) \times (-8) =$

2) $(-4) \times 5 =$

3) $5 \times (-11) =$

4) $(-5) \times (-20) =$

5) $-(2) \times (-8) \times 3 =$

6) $(12 - 4) \times (-10) =$

7) $14 \times (-10) \times (-5) =$

8) $(18 + 12) \times (-8) =$

9) $9 \times (-15 + 6) \times 3 =$

10) $(-5) \times (-8) \times (-12) =$

✎ **Find each quotient.**

11) $16 \div (-4) =$

12) $(-25) \div (-5) =$

13) $(-40) \div (-8) =$

14) $64 \div (-8) =$

15) $(-49) \div 7 =$

16) $(-112) \div (-4) =$

17) $168 \div (-12) =$

18) $(-121) \div (-11) =$

19) $216 \div (-12) =$

20) $-(152) \div (8) =$

21) $(-152) \div (-8) =$

22) $-216 \div (-12) =$

23) $(-198) \div (-9) =$

24) $195 \div (-13) =$

25) $-(182) \div (-7) =$

26) $(126) \div (-14) =$

Order of Operations

✎ *Evaluate each expression.*

1) $5 + (4 \times 2) =$

2) $13 - (2 \times 5) =$

3) $(16 \times 2) + 18 =$

4) $(12 - 5) - (4 \times 3) =$

5) $25 + (14 \div 2) =$

6) $(18 \times 5) \div 5 =$

7) $(48 \div 2) \times (-4) =$

8) $(7 \times 5) + (25 - 12) =$

9) $64 + (3 \times 2) + 8 =$

10) $(20 \times 5) \div (4 + 1) =$

11) $(-9) + (12 \times 6) + 15 =$

12) $(7 \times 8) - (56 \div 4) =$

13) $(4 \times 8 \div 2) - (17 + 11) =$

14) $(18 + 8 - 15) \times 5 - 3 =$

15) $(25 - 12 + 45) \times (95 \div 5) =$

16) $28 + (15 - (32 \div 2)) =$

17) $(6 + 7 - 4 - 9) + (18 \div 2) =$

18) $(95 - 17) + (10 - 25 + 9) =$

19) $(18 \times 2) + (15 \times 5) - 12 =$

20) $12 + 8 - (42 \times 4) + 50 =$

Ordering Integers and Numbers

✎ **Order each set of integers from least to greatest.**

1) $7, -9, -6, -1, 3$ ___, ___, ___, ___, ___, ___

2) $-4, -11, 5, 12, 9$ ___, ___, ___, ___, ___, ___

3) $18, -12, -19, 21, -20$ ___, ___, ___, ___, ___, ___

4) $-15, -25, 18, -7, 32$ ___, ___, ___, ___, ___, ___

5) $37, -42, 28, -11, 34$ ___, ___, ___, ___, ___, ___

6) $78, 46, -19, 77, -24$ ___, ___, ___, ___, ___, ___

✎ **Order each set of integers from greatest to least.**

7) $11, 16, -9, -12, -4$ ___, ___, ___, ___, ___, ___

8) $23, 31, -14, -20, 39$ ___, ___, ___, ___, ___, ___

9) $45, -21, -18, 55, -5$ ___, ___, ___, ___, ___, ___

10) $68, 81, -14, -10, 94$ ___, ___, ___, ___, ___, ___

11) $-5, 69, -12, -43, 34$ ___, ___, ___, ___, ___, ___

12) $-56, -25, -30, 18, 29$ ___, ___, ___, ___, ___, ___

Integers and Absolute Value

✎ **Write absolute value of each number.**

1) $|-7| =$

2) $|-11| =$

3) $|-9| =$

4) $|8| =$

5) $|4| =$

6) $|-18| =$

7) $|6| =$

8) $|0| =$

9) $|16| =$

10) $|-2| =$

11) $|-12|$

12) $|10| =$

13) $|3| =$

14) $|7| =$

15) $|-15| =$

16) $|-13| =$

17) $|19| =$

18) $|-12| =$

19) $|4| =$

20) $|-25| =$

✎ **Evaluate the value.**

21) $|-2| - \frac{|-10|}{2} =$

22) $8 - |2 - 14| - |-2| =$

23) $\frac{|-36|}{6} \times |-6| =$

24) $\frac{|5 \times -3|}{5} \times \frac{|-2|}{4} =$

25) $|2 \times -4| + \frac{|-40|}{5} =$

26) $\frac{|-28|}{4} \times \frac{|-55|}{11} =$

27) $|-12 + 4| \times \frac{|-4 \times 5|}{2}$

28) $\frac{|-10 \times 3|}{2} \times |-12| =$

Answers of Worksheets – Chapter 2

Adding and Subtracting Integers

1) 7
2) -32
3) -20
4) 31
5) -14
6) 33
7) 16
8) 3
9) 5
10) 37
11) -4
12) 35
13) -36
14) 46
15) 34
16) 53
17) 93
18) 11
19) 26
20) 71
21) 38
22) 9
23) -11
24) -1
25) 49
26) 11

Multiplying and Dividing Integers

1) 56
2) -20
3) -55
4) 100
5) 48
6) -80
7) 700
8) -240
9) -243
10) -480
11) -4
12) 5
13) 5
14) -8
15) -7
16) 28
17) -14
18) 11
19) -18
20) -19
21) 19
22) 18
23) 22
24) -15
25) 26
26) -9

Order of Operations

1) 13
2) 3
3) 50
4) -5
5) 32
6) 18
7) -96
8) 48
9) 78
10) 20
11) 78
12) 42
13) -12
14) 52
15) 1,102
16) 27
17) 9
18) 72
19) 99
20) -98

Ordering Integers and Numbers

1) $-9, -6, -1, 3, 7$
2) $-11, -4, 5, 9, 12$
3) $-20, -19, -12, 18, 21$
4) $-25, -15, -7, 18, 32$
5) $-42, -11, 28, 34, 37$
6) $-24, -19, 46, 77, 78$

7) 16, 11, −4, −9, −12
8) 39, 31, 23, −14, −20
9) 55, 45, −5, −18, −21
10) 94, 81, 68, −10, −14
11) 69, 34, −5, −12, −43
12) 29, 18, −25, −30, −56

Integers and Absolute Value

1) 7
2) 11
3) 9
4) 8
5) 4
6) 18
7) 6
8) 0
9) 16
10) 2
11) 12
12) 10
13) 3
14) 7
15) 15
16) 13
17) 19
18) 12
19) 4
20) 25
21) −3
22) −6
23) 36
24) 15
25) 16
26) 35
27) 80
28) 180

Chapter 3:

Proportions, Ratios, and Percent

Topics that you'll practice in this chapter:

✓ Simplifying Ratios

✓ Proportional Ratios

✓ Similarity and Ratios

✓ Ratio and Rates Word Problems

✓ Percentage Calculations

✓ Percent Problems

✓ Discount, Tax and Tip

✓ Percent of Change

✓ Simple Interest

Without Math, there's nothing you can do. Everything around you is Mathematics. Everything around you is numbers." – Shakuntala Devi

Simplifying Ratios

✎ Reduce each ratio.

1) $12:8 =$ ___ : ___
2) $2:20 =$ ___ : ___
3) $3:36 =$ ___ : ___
4) $8:16 =$ ___ : ___
5) $6:100 =$ ___ : ___
6) $10:60 =$ ___ : ___
7) $21:49 =$ ___ : ___
8) $20:40 =$ ___ : ___

9) $10:50 =$ ___ : ___
10) $14:18 =$ ___ : ___
11) $45:27 =$ ___ : ___
12) $49:21 =$ ___ : ___
13) $100:10 =$ ___ : ___
14) $35:45 =$ ___ : ___
15) $8:20 =$ ___ : ___
16) $25:35 =$ ___ : ___

17) $21:27 =$ ___ : ___
18) $52:82 =$ ___ : ___
19) $12:36 =$ ___ : ___
20) $24:3 =$ ___ : ___
21) $15:30 =$ ___ : ___
22) $14:63 =$ ___ : ___
23) $68:80 =$ ___ : ___
24) $8:80 =$ ___ : ___

✎ Write each ratio as a fraction in simplest form.

25) $2:4 =$
26) $6:20 =$
27) $5:35 =$
28) $10:55 =$
29) $8:24 =$
30) $9:42 =$
31) $12:48 =$

32) $6:40 =$
33) $15:36 =$
34) $18:82 =$
35) $22:26 =$
36) $8:36 =$
37) $16:128 =$
38) $14:77 =$

39) $12:180 =$
40) $36:108 =$
41) $24:42 =$
42) $18:120 =$
43) $44:82 =$
44) $60:240 =$
45) $36:180 =$

Proportional Ratios

✎ *Fill in the blanks; solve each proportion.*

1) $3 : 7 \ = \ \_\_ : 49$

2) $1 : 2 \ = \ 20 : \_\_$

3) $1 : 5 \ = \ \_\_ : 50$

4) $7 : 9 \ = \ 14 : \_\_$

5) $5 : 3 \ = \ 45 : \_\_$

6) $7 : 3 \ = \ \_\_ : 18$

7) $10 : 1 \ = \ \_\_ : 10$

8) $1 : 3 \ = \ \_\_ : 27$

9) $8 : 1 \ = \ \_\_ : 8$

10) $9 : 2 \ = \ \_\_ : 14$

11) $3 : 12 \ = \ 12 : \_\_$

12) $6 : 4 \ = \ 24 : \_\_$

✎ *State if each pair of ratios form a proportion.*

13) $\frac{3}{10}$ and $\frac{9}{30}$

14) $\frac{1}{2}$ and $\frac{16}{32}$

15) $\frac{5}{6}$ and $\frac{35}{42}$

16) $\frac{3}{7}$ and $\frac{27}{72}$

17) $\frac{2}{5}$ and $\frac{16}{45}$

18) $\frac{4}{9}$ and $\frac{40}{81}$

19) $\frac{6}{11}$ and $\frac{42}{77}$

20) $\frac{1}{6}$ and $\frac{8}{48}$

21) $\frac{6}{17}$ and $\frac{36}{85}$

22) $\frac{2}{7}$ and $\frac{24}{86}$

23) $\frac{12}{19}$ and $\frac{156}{247}$

24) $\frac{13}{21}$ and $\frac{182}{294}$

✎ *Solve each proportion.*

25) $\frac{2}{5} = \frac{14}{x}, x = \_\_\_\_$

26) $\frac{1}{6} = \frac{7}{x}, x = \_\_\_\_$

27) $\frac{3}{5} = \frac{27}{x}, x = \_\_\_\_$

28) $\frac{1}{5} = \frac{x}{80}, x = \_\_\_\_$

29) $\frac{3}{7} = \frac{x}{63}, x = \_\_\_\_$

30) $\frac{1}{4} = \frac{13}{x}, x = \_\_\_\_$

31) $\frac{7}{9} = \frac{56}{x}, x = \_\_\_\_$

32) $\frac{6}{11} = \frac{42}{x}, x = \_\_\_\_$

33) $\frac{4}{7} = \frac{x}{77}, x = \_\_\_\_$

34) $\frac{5}{13} = \frac{x}{143}, x = \_\_\_\_$

35) $\frac{7}{19} = \frac{x}{209}, x = \_\_\_\_$

36) $\frac{3}{13} = \frac{x}{195}, x = \_\_\_\_$

Similarity and Ratios

✏️ *Each pair of figures is similar. Find the missing side.*

1)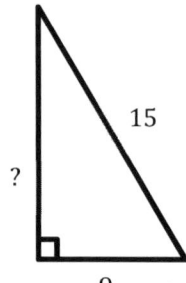

2)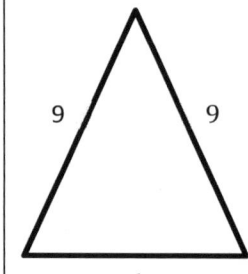

3)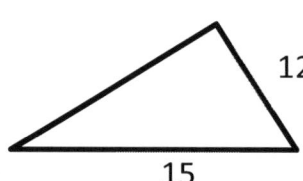

4)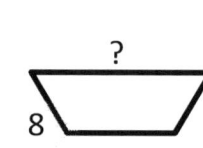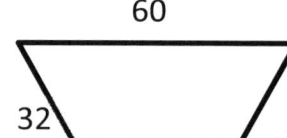

✏️ *Solve.*

5) Two rectangles are similar. The first is 6 feet wide and 20 feet long. The second is 15 feet wide. What is the length of the second rectangle? _____

6) Two rectangles are similar. One is 2.5 meters by 9 meters. The longer side of the second rectangle is 22.5 meters. What is the other side of the second rectangle? _____

7) A building casts a shadow 24 ft long. At the same time a girl 5 ft tall casts a shadow 2 ft long. How tall is the building? _____

8) The scale of a map of Texas is 2 inches: 45 miles. If you measure the distance from Dallas to Martin County as 14.4 inches, approximately how far is Martin County from Dallas? _____

Ratio and Rates Word Problems

✍ **Solve each word problem.**

1) Bob has 12 red cards and 20 green cards. What is the ratio of Bob's red cards to his green cards? _____

2) In a party, 10 soft drinks are required for every 12 guests. If there are 252 guests, how many soft drinks is required? _____

3) In Jack's class, 18 of the students are tall and 10 are short. In Michael's class 54 students are tall and 30 students are short. Which class has a higher ratio of tall to short students? _____

4) The price of 3 apples at the Quick Market is $1.44. The price of 5 of the same apples at Walmart is $2.50. Which place is the better buy? _____

5) The bakers at a Bakery can make 160 bagels in 4 hours. How many bagels can they bake in 16 hours? What is that rate per hour? _____

6) You can buy 5 cans of green beans at a supermarket for $3.40. How much does it cost to buy 35 cans of green beans? _____

7) The ratio of boys to girls in a class is 2:3. If there are 18 boys in the class, how many girls are in that class? _____

8) The ratio of red marbles to blue marbles in a bag is 3:4. If there are 42 marbles in the bag, how many of the marbles are red? _____

Percentage Calculations

✎ **Calculate the given percent of each value.**

1) 2% of 50 = ____
2) 10% of 30 = ____
3) 20% of 25 = ____
4) 50% of 80 = ____
5) 40% of 200 = ____
6) 20% of 45 = ____

7) 35% of 20 = ____
8) 12% of 400 = ____
9) 40% of 90 = ____
10) 25% of 812 = ____
11) 32% of 600 = ____
12) 87% of 500 = ____

13) 77% of 300 = ____
14) 29% of 86 = ____
15) 33% of 54 = ____
16) 71% of 112 = ____
17) 44% of 165 = ____
18) 17% of 232 = ____

✎ **Calculate the percent of each given value.**

19) ____% of 7 = 3.5
20) ____% of 15 = 9
21) ____% of 80 = 4
22) ____% of 50 = 12.5
23) ____% of 64 = 8

24) ____% of 72 = 18
25) ____% of 250 = 12.5
26) ____% of 400 = 12
27) ____% of 190 = 9.5
28) ____% of 900 = 126

✎ **Solve each percent problem.**

29) A Cinema has 240 seats. 144 seats were sold for the current movie. What percent of seats are empty? _____ %

30) There are 18 boys and 46 girls in a class. 87.5% of the students in the class take the bus to school. How many students do not take the bus to school? _____

Percent Problems

✍ **Solve each problem.**

1) 20 is what percent of 50? ____%

2) 18 is what percent of 90? ____%

3) 12 is what percent of 15? ____%

4) 16 is what percent of 200? ____%

5) 24 is what percent of 800? ____%

6) 48 is what percent of 4,00? ____%

7) 90 is what percent of 750? ____%

8) 24 is what percent of 300? ____%

9) 60 is what percent of 400? ____%

10) 42 is what percent of 350? ___%

11) 11 is what percent of 44? ___%

12) 8 is what percent of 64? ___%

13) 210 is what percent of 875? ___%

14) 80 is what percent of 64? ___%

15) 15 is what percent of 12? ___%

16) 56 is what percent of 40? ___%

17) 36 is what percent of 240? ___%

18) 32 is what percent of 20? ___%

✍ **Solve each percent word problem.**

19) There are 48 employees in a company. On a certain day, 36 were present. What percent showed up for work? _____%

20) A metal bar weighs 24 ounces. 15% of the bar is gold. How many ounces of gold are in the bar? _____

21) A crew is made up of 12 women; the rest are men. If 20% of the crew are women, how many people are in the crew? _____

22) There are 48 students in a class and 6 of them are girls. What percent are boys? _____%

23) The Royals softball team played 75 games and won 60 of them. What percent of the games did they lose? _____%

Discount, Tax and Tip

✎ *Find the selling price of each item.*

1) Original price of a computer: $500
   Tax: 6%   Selling price: $_____

2) Original price of a laptop: $350
   Tax: 8%   Selling price: $_____

3) Original price of a sofa: $800
   Tax: 7%   Selling price: $_____

4) Original price of a car: $18,500
   Tax: 8.5%   Selling price: $_____

5) Original price of a Table: $250
   Tax: 5%   Selling price: $_____

6) Original price of a house: $250,000
   Tax: 6.5%   Selling price: $_____

7) Original price of a tablet: $400
   Discount: 20%   Selling price: $_____

8) Original price of a chair: $150
   Discount: 15%   Selling price: $_____

9) Original price of a book: $50
   Discount: 25%   Selling price: $_____

10) Original price of a cellphone: $500
    Discount: 10%   Selling price: $_____

11) Food bill: $24
    Tip: 20%   Price: $_____

12) Food bill: $60
    Tipp: 15%   Price: $_____

13) Food bill: $32
    Tip: 20%   Price: $_____

14) Food bill: $18
    Tipp: 25%   Price: $_____

✎ *Solve each word problem.*

15) Nicolas hired a moving company. The company charDAT $400 for its services, and Nicolas gives the movers a 15% tip. How much does Nicolas tip the movers? $_____

16) Mason has lunch at a restaurant and the cost of his meal is $30. Mason wants to leave a 20% tip. What is Mason's total bill including tip? $_____

17) The sales tax in Texas is 8.25% and an item costs $400. How much is the tax? $_____

18) The price of a table at Best Buy is $220. If the sales tax is 6%, what is the final price of the table including tax? $_____

Percent of Change

✎ **Find each percent of change.**

1) From 200 to 500. ___ %

2) From 50 ft to 75 ft. ___ %

3) From $250 to $350. ___ %

4) From 60 cm to 90 cm. ___ %

5) From 30 to 90. ___ %

6) From 30 to 6. ___ %

7) From 80 to 120. ___ %

8) From 800 to 200. ___ %

9) From 25 to 15. ___ %

10) From 32 to 8. ___ %

✎ **Solve each percent of change word problem.**

11) Bob got a raise, and his hourly wage increased from $12 to $15. What is the percent increase? _____ %

12) The price of a pair of shoes increases from $20 to $32. What is the percent increase? ___ %

13) At a coffeeshop, the price of a cup of coffee increased from $1.20 to $1.44. What is the percent increase in the cost of the coffee? _____ %

14) 6 cm are cut from a 24 cm board. What is the percent decrease in length? _____ %

15) In a class, the number of students has been increased from 18 to 27. What is the percent increase? _____ %

16) The price of gasoline rose from $2.40 to $2.76 in one month. By what percent did the gas price rise? _____ %

17) A shirt was originally priced at $48. It went on sale for $38.40. What was the percent that the shirt was discounted? _____ %

Simple Interest

✎ *Determine the simple interest for these loans.*

1) $450 at 7% for 2 years. $ _____
2) $5,200 at 4% for 3 years. $ _____
3) $1,300 at 5% for 6 years. $ _____
4) $5,400 at 3.5% for 6 months. $ _____
5) $600 at 4% for 9 months. $ _____

6) $24,000 at 5.5% for 5 years. $ _____
7) $15,600 at 3% for 2 years. $ _____
8) $1,200 at 5.5% for 4 years. $ _____
9) $1,600 at 4.5 % for 9 months. $ _____
10) $12,000 at 2.2% for 5 years. $ _____

✎ *Solve each simple interest word problem.*

11) A new car, valued at $28,000, depreciates at 9% per year. What is the value of the car one year after purchase? $ _____

12) Sara puts $4,000 into an investment yielding 5% annual simple interest; she left the money in for five years. How much interest does Sara get at the end of those five years? $ _____

13) A bank is offering 3.5% simple interest on a savings account. If you deposit $7,500, how much interest will you earn in two years? $ _____

14) $400 interest is earned on a principal of $2,000 at a simple interest rate of 5% interest per year. For how many years was the principal invested? _____

15) In how many years will $1,200 yield an interest of $180 at 3% simple interest? _____

16) Jim invested $4,000 in a bond at a yearly rate of 4.5%. He earned $540 in interest. How long was the money invested? _____

Answers of Worksheets – Chapter 3

Simplifying Ratios

1) 3 : 2
2) 1 : 10
3) 1 : 12
4) 1 : 2
5) 3 : 50
6) 1 : 6
7) 3 : 7
8) 1 : 2
9) 1 : 5
10) 7 : 9
11) 5 : 3
12) 7 : 3
13) 10 : 1
14) 7 : 9
15) 2 : 5
16) 5 : 7
17) 7 : 9
18) 26 : 41
19) 1 : 3
20) 8 : 1
21) 1 : 2
22) 2 : 9
23) 17 : 20
24) 1 : 10
25) $\frac{1}{2}$
26) $\frac{3}{10}$
27) $\frac{1}{7}$
28) $\frac{2}{11}$
29) $\frac{1}{3}$
30) $\frac{3}{14}$
31) $\frac{1}{4}$
32) $\frac{3}{20}$
33) $\frac{5}{12}$
34) $\frac{9}{41}$
35) $\frac{11}{13}$
36) $\frac{2}{9}$
37) $\frac{1}{8}$
38) $\frac{2}{11}$
39) $\frac{1}{15}$
40) $\frac{1}{3}$
41) $\frac{4}{7}$
42) $\frac{3}{20}$
43) $\frac{22}{41}$
44) $\frac{1}{4}$
45) $\frac{1}{5}$

Proportional Ratios

1) 21
2) 40
3) 10
4) 18
5) 27
6) 42
7) 100
8) 9
9) 64
10) 63
11) 48
12) 16
13) Yes
14) Yes
15) Yes
16) No
17) No
18) No
19) Yes
20) Yes
21) No
22) No
23) Yes
24) Yes
25) 35
26) 42
27) 45
28) 16
29) 27
30) 52
31) 72
32) 77
33) 44
34) 55
35) 77
36) 45

Similarity and ratios

1) 12
2) 2
3) 5
4) 15
5) 50 feet
6) 6.25 meters
7) 60 feet
8) 324 miles

Ratio and Rates Word Problems

1) 3 : 5
2) 210
3) The ratio for both classes is 9 to 5.
4) Quick Market is a better buy.
5) 640, the rate is 40 per hour.
6) $23.80
7) 27
8) 18

Percentage Calculations

1) 1
2) 3
3) 5
4) 40
5) 80
6) 9
7) 7
8) 48
9) 36
10) 203
11) 192
12) 435
13) 231
14) 24.94
15) 17.82
16) 79.52
17) 72.6
18) 39.44
19) 50%
20) 60%
21) 5%
22) 25%
23) 12.5%
24) 25%
25) 5%
26) 3%
27) 5%
28) 14%
29) 40%
30) 8

Percent Problems

1) 40%
2) 20%
3) 80%
4) 8%
5) 3%
6) 12%
7) 12%
8) 8%
9) 15%
10) 12%
11) 25%
12) 12.5%
13) 24%
14) 125%
15) 125%
16) 140%
17) 15%
18) 160%
19) 75%
20) 3.6 ounces
21) 60
22) 87.5%
23) 20%

Discount, Tax and Tip

1) $530.00
2) $378.00
3) $856.00
4) $20,072.50
5) $262.50
6) $266,250
7) $320.00
8) $127.50
9) $37.50

10) $450.00	13) $38.40	16) $36.00
11) $28.80	14) $22.50	17) $33.00
12) $69.00	15) $60.00	18) $233.20

Percent of Change

1) 150%	7) 50%	13) 20%
2) 50%	8) 75%	14) 25%
3) 40%	9) 40%	15) 50%
4) 50%	10) 75%	16) 15%
5) 200%	11) 25%	17) 20%
6) 80%	12) 60%	

Simple Interest

1) $63.00	7) $936.00	13) $525.00
2) $624.00	8) $264.00	14) 4 years
3) $390.00	9) $54	15) 5 years
4) $94.50	10) $1,320.00	16) 3 years
5) $18.00	11) $25,480.00	
6) $6,600.00	12) $1,000.00	

Chapter 4:

Algebraic Expressions

Topics that you'll practice in this chapter:

✓ Simplifying Variable Expressions

✓ Simplifying Polynomial Expressions

✓ Translate Phrases into an Algebraic Statement

✓ The Distributive Property

✓ Evaluating One Variable Expressions

✓ Evaluating Two Variables Expressions

✓ Combining like Terms

Mathematics is, as it were, a sensuous logic, and relates to philosophy as do the arts, music, and plastic art to poetry. — K. Shegel

Simplifying Variable Expressions

✏️ *Simplify each expression.*

1) $3(x + 9) =$

2) $(-6)(8x - 4) =$

3) $7x + 3 - 3x =$

4) $-2 - x^2 - 6x^2 =$

5) $3 + 10x^2 + 2 =$

6) $8x^2 + 6x + 7x^2 =$

7) $5x^2 - 12x^2 + 8x =$

8) $2x^2 - 2x - x =$

9) $4x + 6(2 - 5x) =$

10) $10x + 8(10x - 6) =$

11) $9(-2x - 6) - 5 =$

12) $2x^2 + (-8x) =$

13) $x - 3 + 5 - 3x =$

14) $2 - 3x + 12 - 2x =$

15) $32x - 4 + 23 + 2x =$

16) $(-6)(8x - 4) + 10x =$

17) $14x - 5(5 - 8x) =$

18) $23x + 4(9x + 3) + 12 =$

19) $3(-7x + 5) + 20x =$

20) $12x - 3x(x + 9) =$

21) $7x + 5x(3 - 3x) =$

22) $5x(-8x + 12) + 14x =$

23) $40x + 12 + 2x^2 =$

24) $5x(x - 3) - 10 =$

25) $8x - 7 + 8x + 2x^2 =$

26) $2x^2 - 5x - 7x =$

27) $7x - 3x^2 - 5x^2 - 3 =$

28) $4 + x^2 - 6x^2 - 12x =$

29) $12x + 8x^2 + 2x + 20 =$

30) $2x^2 + 6x + 3x^2 =$

31) $23 + 15x^2 + 8x - 4x^2 =$

32) $8x - 12x - x^2 + 13 =$

Simplifying Polynomial Expressions

✎ **Simplify each polynomial.**

1) $(2x^3 + 5x^2) - (12x + 2x^2) =$ _____

2) $(2x^5 + 2x^3) - (7x^3 + 6x^2) =$ _____

3) $(12x^4 + 4x^2) - (2x^2 - 6x^4) =$ _____

4) $14x - 3x^2 - 2(6x^2 + 6x^3) =$ _____

5) $(5x^3 - 3) + 5(2x^2 - 3x^3) =$ _____

6) $(4x^3 - 2x) - 2(4x^3 - 2x^4) =$ _____

7) $2(4x - 3x^3) - 3(3x^3 + 4x^2) =$ _____

8) $(2x^2 - 2x) - (2x^3 + 5x^2) =$ _____

9) $2x^3 - (4x^4 + 2x) + x^2 =$ _____

10) $x^4 - 2(x^2 + x) + 3x =$ _____

11) $(2x^2 - x^4) - (4x^4 - x^2) =$ _____

12) $4x^2 - 5x^3 + 15x^4 - 12x^3 =$ _____

13) $2x^2 - 5x^4 + 14x^4 - 11x^3 =$ _____

14) $2x^2 + 5x^3 - 7x^2 + 12x =$ _____

15) $2x^4 - 5x^5 + 8x^4 - 8x^2 =$ _____

16) $5x^3 + 15x - x^2 - 2x^3 =$ _____

Translate Phrases into an Algebraic Statement

✎ *Write an algebraic expression for each phrase.*

1) 4 multiplied by x. _____

2) Subtract 8 from y. _____

3) 6 divided by x. _____

4) 12 decreased by y. _____

5) Add y to 9. _____

6) The square of 5. _____

7) x raised to the fourth power. _____

8) The sum of nine and a number. _____

9) The difference between sixty–four and y. _____

10) The quotient of twelve and a number. _____

11) The quotient of the square of x and 7. _____

12) The difference between x and 8 is 22. _____

13) 2 times a reduced by the square of b. _____

14) Subtract the product of a and b from 12. _____

The Distributive Property

✍ **Use the distributive property to simply each expression.**

1) $2(2 + 3x) =$

2) $3(5 + 5x) =$

3) $4(3x - 8) =$

4) $(6x - 2)(-2) =$

5) $(-3)(x + 2) =$

6) $(2 + 2x)5 =$

7) $(-4)(4 - 2x) =$

8) $-(-2 - 5x) =$

9) $(-6x + 2)(-1) =$

10) $(-5)(x - 2) =$

11) $-(7 - 3x) =$

12) $8(8 + 2x) =$

13) $2(12 + 2x) =$

14) $(-6x + 8)4 =$

15) $(3 - 6x)(-7) =$

16) $(-12)(2x + 1) =$

17) $(8 - 2x)9 =$

18) $5(7 + 9x) =$

19) $11(5x + 2) =$

20) $(-4x + 6)6 =$

21) $(3 - 6x)(-8) =$

22) $(-12)(2x - 3) =$

23) $(10 - 2x)9 =$

24) $(-5)(11x - 2) =$

25) $(1 - 9x)(-10) =$

26) $(-6)(x + 8) =$

27) $(-4 + 3x)(-8) =$

28) $(-5)(1 - 11x) =$

29) $11(3x - 12) =$

30) $(-12x + 14)(-5) =$

31) $(-5)(4x - 1) + 4(x + 2) =$

32) $(-3)(x + 4) - (2 + 3x) =$

Evaluating One Variable Expressions

✎ *Evaluate each expression using the value given.*

1) $5 + x$, $x = 2$

2) $x - 2$, $x = 4$

3) $8x + 1$, $x = 9$

4) $x - 12$, $x = -1$

5) $9 - x$, $x = 3$

6) $x + 2$, $x = 5$

7) $3x + 7$, $x = 6$

8) $x + (-5)$, $x = -2$

9) $3x + 6$, $x = 4$

10) $4x + 6$, $x = -1$

11) $10 + 2x - 6$, $x = 3$

12) $10 - 3x$, $x = 8$

13) $2x - 5$, $x = 4$

14) $5x + 6$, $x = -3$

15) $12x + 6$, $x = 2$

16) $10 - 3x$, $x = -2$

17) $5(6x + 2)$, $x = 8$

18) $2(-7x - 2)$, $x = 3$

19) $9x - 3x + 12$, $x = 6$

20) $(6x + 3) \div 5$, $x = 2$

21) $(x + 16) \div 3$, $x = 8$

22) $4x - 12 + 8x$, $x = -6$

23) $(16 - 12x)(-2)$, $x = -3$

24) $12x^2 + 5x - 3$, $x = 2$

25) $x^2 - 11x$, $x = -4$

26) $2x(6 - 4x)$, $x = 5$

27) $14x + 7 - 3x^2$, $x = -3$

28) $(-5)(10x - 20 + 2x)$, $x = 2$

29) $(-3) + \frac{x}{4} + 2x$, $x = 16$

30) $(-2) + \frac{x}{7}$, $x = 21$

31) $\left(-\frac{14}{x}\right) - 9 + 4x$, $x = 2$

32) $\left(-\frac{6}{x}\right) - 9 + 2x$, $x = 3$

Evaluating Two Variables Expressions

✎ *Evaluate each expression using the values given.*

1) $2x + 4y$,
   $x = 3, y = 2$

2) $8x + 5y$,
   $x = 1, y = 5$

3) $-2a + 4b$,
   $a = 6, b = 3$

4) $4x + 7 - 2y$,
   $x = 7, y = 6$

5) $5z + 12 - 4k$,
   $z = 5, k = 2$

6) $2(-x - 2y)$,
   $x = 6, y = 9$

7) $18a + 2b$,
   $a = 2, b = 8$

8) $4x \div 3y$,
   $x = 3, y = 2$

9) $2x + 15 + 4y$,
   $x = -2, y = 4$

10) $4a - (15 - b)$,
    $a = 4, b = 6$

11) $5z + 19 + 8k$,
    $z = -5, k = 4$

12) $xy + 12 + 5x$,
    $x = 7, y = 2$

13) $2x + 4y - 3 + 2$,
    $x = 5, y = 3$

14) $\left(-\frac{12}{x}\right) + 1 + 5y$,
    $x = 6, y = 8$

15) $(-4)(-2a - 2b)$,
    $a = 5, b = 3$

16) $10 + 3x + 7 - 2y$,
    $x = 7, y = 6$

17) $9x + 2 - 4y + 5$,
    $x = 7, y = 5$

18) $6 + 3(-2x - 3y)$,
    $x = 9, y = 7$

19) $2x + 14 + 4y$,
    $x = 6, y = 8$

20) $4a - (5a - b) + 5$,
    $a = 4, b = 6$

Combining like Terms

✎ *Simplify each expression.*

1) $2x + x + 2 =$

2) $2(5x - 3) =$

3) $7x - 2x + 8 =$

4) $(-4)(3x - 5) =$

5) $9x - 7x - 5 =$

6) $16x - 5 + 8x =$

7) $5 - (5x + 6) =$

8) $-12x + 7 - 10x =$

9) $7x - 11 - 2x + 2 =$

10) $12x + 4x - 21 =$

11) $5 + 2x - 8 =$

12) $(-2x + 6)2 =$

13) $7 + 3x + 6x - 4 =$

14) $9(x - 7x) - 5 =$

15) $7(3x + 6) + 2x =$

16) $3x - 12 - 5x =$

17) $2(4 + 3x) - 7x =$

18) $22x + 6 + 2x =$

19) $(-5x) + 12 + 7x =$

20) $(-3x) - 9 + 15x =$

21) $2(5x + 7) + 8x =$

22) $2(9 - 3x) - 17x =$

23) $-4x - (6 - 14x) =$

24) $(-4) - (3)(5x + 8) =$

25) $(-2)(9x - 3) - 12x =$

26) $-22x + 6 + 4x - 3x =$

27) $4(-13x + 2) - 14x =$

28) $-6x - 19 + 15x =$

29) $21x - 12x + 6 - 7x =$

30) $5(6x + 2x) - 15 =$

31) $18 - 12x - 25 - 15x =$

32) $-3(-4x - 2x) + 8x =$

Answers of Worksheets – Chapter 4

Simplifying Variable Expressions

1) $3x + 27$
2) $-48x + 24$
3) $4x + 3$
4) $-7x^2 - 2$
5) $10x^2 + 5$
6) $15x^2 + 6x$
7) $-7x^2 + 8x$
8) $2x^2 - 3x$
9) $-24x + 12$
10) $90x - 48$
11) $-18x - 59$
12) $2x^2 - 8x$
13) $-2x + 2$
14) $-5x + 14$
15) $34x + 19$
16) $-38x + 24$
17) $54x - 25$
18) $59x + 24$
19) $-x + 15$
20) $-3x^2 - 15x$
21) $-15x^2 + 22x$
22) $-40x^2 + 74x$
23) $2x^2 + 40x + 12$
24) $5x^2 - 15x - 10$
25) $2x^2 + 16x - 7$
26) $2x^2 - 12x$
27) $-8x^2 + 7x - 3$
28) $-5x^2 - 12x + 4$
29) $8x^2 + 14x + 20$
30) $5x^2 + 6x$
31) $11x^2 + 8x + 23$
32) $-x^2 - 4x + 13$

Simplifying Polynomial Expressions

1) $2x^3 + 3x^2 - 12x$
2) $2x^5 - 5x^3 - 6x^2$
3) $18x^4 + 2x^2$
4) $-12x^3 - 15x^2 + 14x$
5) $-10x^3 + 10x^2 - 3$
6) $4x^4 - 4x^3 - 2x$
7) $-15x^3 - 12x^2 + 8x$
8) $-2x^3 - 3x^2 - 2x$
9) $-4x^4 + 2x^3 + x^2 - 2x$
10) $x^4 - 2x^2 + x$
11) $-5x^4 + 3x^2$
12) $15x^4 - 17x^3 + 4x^2$
13) $9x^4 - 11x^3 + 2x^2$
14) $5x^3 - 5x^2 + 12x$
15) $-5x^5 + 10x^4 - 8x^2$
16) $3x^3 - x^2 + 15x$

Translate Phrases into an Algebraic Statement

1) $4x$
2) $y - 8$
3) $\frac{6}{x}$
4) $12 - y$
5) $y + 9$
6) 5^2
7) x^4
8) $9 + x$
9) $64 - y$
10) $\frac{12}{x}$
11) $\frac{x^2}{7}$
12) $x - 8 = 22$
13) $2a - b^2$
14) $12 - ab$

The Distributive Property

1) $6x + 4$
2) $15x + 15$
3) $12x - 32$
4) $-12x + 4$
5) $-3x - 6$
6) $10x + 10$
7) $8x - 16$
8) $5x + 2$
9) $6x - 2$
10) $-5x + 10$
11) $3x - 7$
12) $16x + 64$
13) $4x + 24$
14) $-24x + 32$
15) $42x - 21$
16) $-24x - 12$
17) $-18x + 72$
18) $45x + 35$
19) $55x + 22$
20) $-24x + 36$
21) $48x - 24$
22) $-24x + 36$
23) $-18x + 90$
24) $-55x + 10$

25) $90x - 10$
26) $-6x - 48$
27) $-24x + 32$
28) $55x - 5$
29) $33x - 132$
30) $60x - 70$
31) $-16x + 13$
32) $-6x - 14$

Evaluating One Variables

1) 7
2) 2
3) 73
4) −13
5) 6
6) 7
7) 25
8) −7
9) 18
10) 2
11) 10
12) −14
13) 3
14) −9
15) 30
16) 16
17) 250
18) −46
19) 48
20) 3
21) 8
22) −84
23) −104
24) 55
25) 60
26) −140
27) −62
28) −20
29) 33
30) 1
31) −8
32) −5

Evaluating Two Variables

1) 14
2) 33
3) 0
4) 23
5) 29
6) −48
7) 52
8) 2
9) 27
10) 7
11) 26
12) 61
13) 21
14) 39
15) 64
16) 26
17) 50
18) −111
19) 58
20) 7

Combining like Terms

1) $3x + 2$
2) $10x - 6$
3) $5x + 8$
4) $-12x + 20$
5) $2x - 5$
6) $24x - 5$
7) $-5x - 1$
8) $-22x + 7$
9) $5x - 9$
10) $16x - 21$
11) $2x - 3$
12) $-4x + 12$
13) $9x + 3$
14) $-54x - 5$
15) $23x + 42$
16) $-2x - 12$
17) $-x + 8$
18) $24x + 6$
19) $2x + 12$
20) $12x - 9$
21) $18x + 14$
22) $-23x + 18$
23) $10x - 6$
24) $-15x - 28$
25) $-30x + 6$
26) $-21x + 6$
27) $-66x + 8$
28) $9x - 19$
29) $2x + 6$
30) $40x - 15$
31) $-27x - 7$
32) $26x$

Chapter 5:

Equations and Inequalities

Topics that you'll practice in this chapter:

✓ One–Step Equations

✓ Multi–Step Equations

✓ Graphing Single–Variable Inequalities

✓ One–Step Inequalities

✓ Multi-Step Inequalities

✓ Systems of Equations

✓ Systems of Equations Word Problems

✓ Quadratic Equations

"Life is a Math equation. In order to gain the most, you have to know how to convert negatives into positives." – Anonymous

One-Step Equations

✍ **Solve each equation.**

1) $2x = 20, x =$ ____

2) $4x = 16, x =$ ____

3) $8x = 24, x =$ ____

4) $6x = 30, x =$ ____

5) $x + 5 = 8, x =$ ____

6) $x - 1 = 5, x =$ ____

7) $x - 8 = 3, x =$ ____

8) $x + 6 = 12, x =$ ____

9) $x - 2 = 17, x =$ ____

10) $8 = 12 + x, x =$ ____

11) $x - 5 = 4, x =$ ____

12) $2 - x = -12, x =$ ____

13) $16 = -4 + x, x =$ ____

14) $x - 4 = -25, x =$ ____

15) $x + 12 = -9, x =$ ____

16) $14 = 18 - x, x =$ ____

17) $2 + x = -14, x =$ ____

18) $x - 5 = 15, x =$ ____

19) $25 = x - 5, x =$ ____

20) $x - 3 = -12, x =$ ____

21) $x - 12 = 12, x =$ ____

22) $x - 12 = -25, x =$ ____

23) $x - 13 = 32, x =$ ____

24) $-55 = x - 18, x =$ ____

25) $x - 12 = 18, x =$ ____

26) $20 = 5x, x =$ ____

27) $x - 30 = 20, x =$ ____

28) $x - 12 = 32, x =$ ____

29) $36 - x = 3, x =$ ____

30) $x - 14 = 14, x =$ ____

31) $19 - x = -15, x =$ ____

32) $x - 19 = -35, x =$ ____

Multi-Step Equations

✎ **Solve each equation.**

1) $2x + 3 = 5$

2) $-x + 8 = 5$

3) $3x - 4 = 5$

4) $-(2 - x) = 5$

5) $2x - 18 = 12$

6) $4x - 2 = 6$

7) $2x - 14 = 4$

8) $5x + 10 = 25$

9) $8x + 9 = 25$

10) $-3(2 + x) = 3$

11) $-2(4 + x) = 4$

12) $20 = -(x - 8)$

13) $2(2 - 2x) = 20$

14) $-12 = -(2x + 8)$

15) $5(2 + x) = 5$

16) $2(x - 14) = 4$

17) $-28 = 2x + 12x$

18) $3x + 15 = -x - 5$

19) $2(3 + 2x) = -18$

20) $12 - 2x = -8 - x$

21) $10 - 3x = 14 + x$

22) $10 + 10x = -2 + 4x$

23) $24 = (-4x) - 8 + 8$

24) $12 = 2x - 12 + 6x$

25) $-12 = -4x - 6 + 2x$

26) $4x - 12 = -18 + 5x$

27) $5x - 10 = 2x + 5$

28) $-7 - 3x = 2(3 - 2x)$

29) $x - 2 = -3(6 - 3x)$

30) $10x - 56 = 12x - 114$

31) $4x - 8 = -4(11 + 2x)$

32) $-5x - 14 = 6x + 52$

Graphing Single–Variable Inequalities

✏️ *Draw a graph for each inequality.*

1) $x > 2$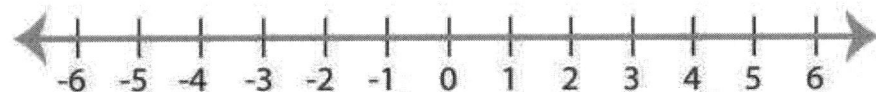

2) $x < 5$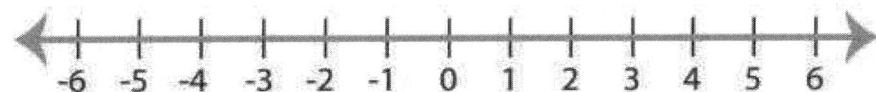

3) $x > -1$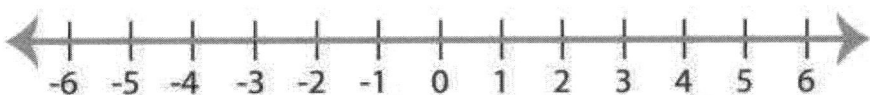

4) $x > 3$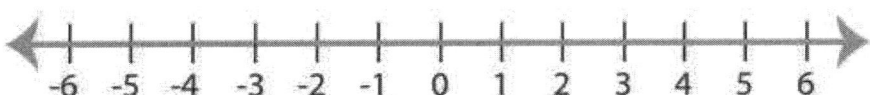

5) $x < -5$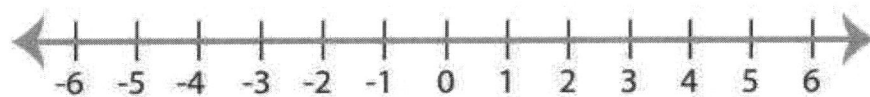

6) $x > -2$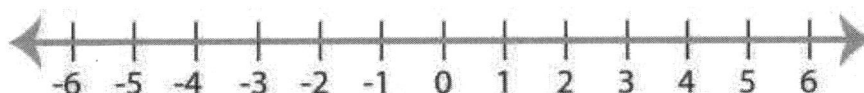

7) $x < 0$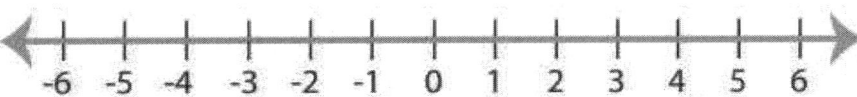

8) $x > 4$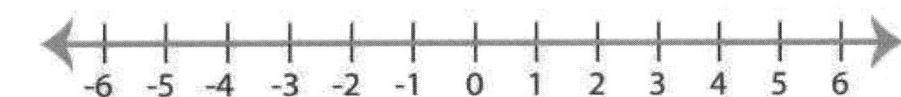

One–Step Inequalities

✎ **Solve each inequality and graph it.**

1) $x + 2 \geq 3$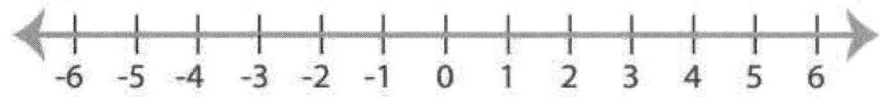

2) $x - 1 \leq 2$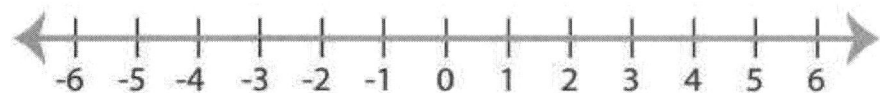

3) $2x \geq 12$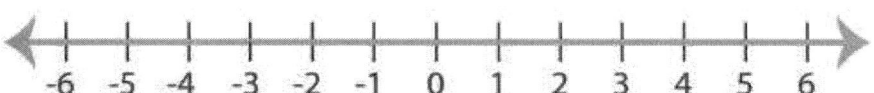

4) $4 + x \leq 5$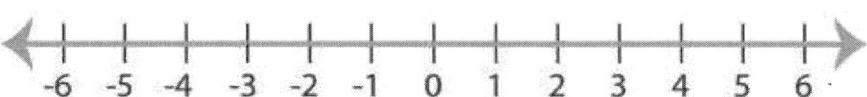

5) $x + 3 \leq -3$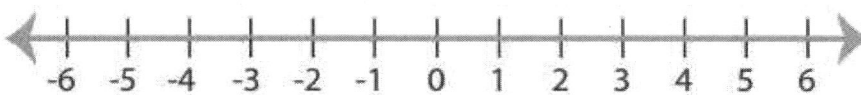

6) $4x \geq 16$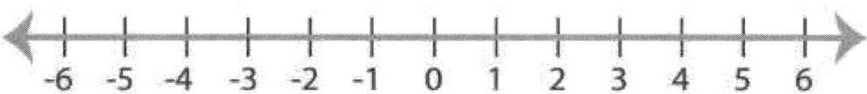

7) $9x \leq 18$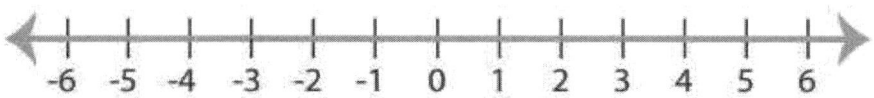

8) $x + 2 \geq 7$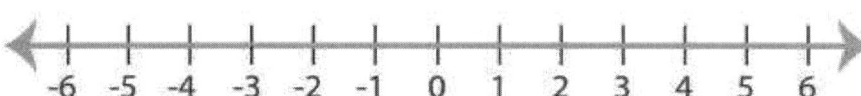

Multi-Step Inequalities

✎ Solve each inequality.

1) $x - 2 \leq 6$

2) $3 - x \leq 3$

3) $2x - 4 \leq 8$

4) $3x - 5 \geq 16$

5) $x - 5 \geq 10$

6) $2x - 8 \leq 6$

7) $8x - 2 \leq 14$

8) $-5 + 3x \leq 10$

9) $2(x - 3) \leq 6$

10) $7x - 5 \leq 9$

11) $4x - 21 < 19$

12) $2x - 3 < 21$

13) $17 - 3x \geq -13$

14) $9 + 4x < 21$

15) $3 + 2x \geq 19$

16) $6 + 2x < 32$

17) $4x - 1 < 7$

18) $3(3 - 2x) \geq -15$

19) $-(3 + 4x) < 13$

20) $20 - 8x \geq -28$

21) $-3(x - 7) > 21$

22) $\dfrac{2x + 6}{4} \leq 10$

23) $\dfrac{4x + 8}{2} \leq 12$

24) $\dfrac{3x - 8}{7} > 1$

25) $4 + \dfrac{x}{3} < 7$

26) $\dfrac{9x}{7} - 7 < 2$

27) $\dfrac{4x + 12}{4} > 1$

28) $15 + \dfrac{x}{5} < 12$

Systems of Equations

✎ **Solve each system of equations.**

1) $-2x + 2y = 4$
   $-2x + y = 3$
   $x = \underline{\quad}$
   $y = \underline{\quad}$

2) $-10x + 2y = -6$
   $6x - 16y = 48$
   $x = \underline{\quad}$
   $y = \underline{\quad}$

3) $y = -8$
   $16x - 12y = 32$
   $x = \underline{\quad}$

4) $2y = -6x + 10$
   $10x - 8y = -6$
   $x = \underline{\quad}$
   $y = \underline{\quad}$

5) $10x - 9y = -13$
   $-5x + 3y = 11$
   $x = \underline{\quad}$
   $y = \underline{\quad}$

6) $-3x - 4y = 5$
   $x - 2y = 5$
   $x = \underline{\quad}$
   $y = \underline{\quad}$

7) $5x - 14y = -23$
   $-6x + 7y = 8$
   $x = \underline{\quad}$
   $y = \underline{\quad}$

8) $10x - 14y = -4$
   $-10x - 20y = -30$
   $x = \underline{\quad}$
   $y = \underline{\quad}$

9) $-4x + 12y = 12$
   $-14x + 16y = -10$
   $x = \underline{\quad}$
   $y = \underline{\quad}$

10) $x + 20y = 56$
    $x + 15y = 41$
    $x = \underline{\quad}$
    $y = \underline{\quad}$

11) $6x - 7y = -8$
    $-x - 4y = -9$
    $x = \underline{\quad}$
    $y = \underline{\quad}$

12) $-3x + 2y = -18$
    $8x - 2y = 28$
    $x = \underline{\quad}$
    $y = \underline{\quad}$

13) $-5x + y = -3$
    $3x - 8y = 24$
    $x = \underline{\quad}$
    $y = \underline{\quad}$

14) $3x - 2y = 2$
    $5x - 5y = 10$
    $x = \underline{\quad}$
    $y = \underline{\quad}$

15) $8x + 14y = 4$
    $-6x - 7y = -10$
    $x = \underline{\quad}$
    $y = \underline{\quad}$

16) $10x + 7y = 1$
    $-5x - 7y = 24$
    $x = \underline{\quad}$
    $y = \underline{\quad}$

Systems of Equations Word Problems

✎ *Solve each word problem.*

1) Tickets to a movie cost $5 for adults and $3 for students. A group of friends purchased 18 tickets for $82.00. How many adults ticket did they buy? _____

2) At a store, Eva bought two shirts and five hats for $154.00. Nicole bought three same shirts and four same hats for $168.00. What is the price of each shirt? _____

3) A farmhouse shelters 10 animals, some are pigs, and some are ducks. Altogether there are 36 legs. How many pigs are there? _____

4) A class of 195 students went on a field trip. They took 19 vehicles, some cars and some buses. If each car holds 5 students and each bus hold 25 students, how many buses did they take? _____

5) A theater is selling tickets for a performance. Mr. Smith purchased 8 senior tickets and 5 child tickets for $136 for his friends and family. Mr. Jackson purchased 4 senior tickets and 6 child tickets for $96. What is the price of a senior ticket? $_____

6) The difference of two numbers is 6. Their sum is 14. What is the bigger number? $_____

7) The sum of the digits of a certain two-digit number is 7. Reversing its digits increase the number by 9. What is the number? _____

8) The difference of two numbers is 18. Their sum is 66. What are the numbers? _____

9) The length of a rectangle is 3 meters greater than 2 times the width. The perimeter of rectangle is 30 meters. What is the length of the rectangle? _____

10) Jim has 44 nickels and dimes totaling $2.95. How many nickels does he have? _____

Quadratic Equation

✎ Multiply.

1) $(x-2)(x+4) = $ _____

2) $(x+1)(x+6) = $ _____

3) $(x-4)(x+2) = $ _____

4) $(x+5)(x-3) = $ _____

5) $(x-6)(x-2) = $ _____

6) $(2x+1)(x-3) = $ _____

7) $(2x-1)(x+4) = $ _____

8) $(2x-3)(x+4) = $ _____

9) $(3x+5)(x-3) = $ _____

10) $(3x+4)(2x-2) = $ _____

✎ Factor each expression.

11) $x^2 - 5x + 4 = $ _____

12) $x^2 + 6x + 8 = $ _____

13) $x^2 + x - 12 = $ _____

14) $x^2 - 7x + 10 = $ _____

15) $x^2 - 4x - 12 = $ _____

16) $2x^2 - 3x - 2 = $ _____

17) $2x^2 + 8x + 8 = $ _____

18) $3x^2 - 14x + 5 = $ _____

19) $3x^2 + 4x + 1 = $ _____

20) $4x^2 - 12x + 8 = $ _____

✎ Solve each equation.

21) $(x+2)(x-4) = 0$

22) $(x+5)(x+8) = 0$

23) $(2x+4)(x+3) = 0$

24) $(3x-9)(2x+6) = 0$

25) $x^2 - 11x + 19 = -5$

26) $x^2 + 7x + 18 = 8$

27) $x^2 - 10x + 22 = -2$

28) $x^2 + 3x - 12 = 6$

29) $5x^2 - 5x - 10 = 0$

30) $6x^2 - 6x = 36$

Answers of Worksheets – Chapter 5

One–Step Equations

1) 10
2) 4
3) 3
4) 5
5) 3
6) 6
7) 11
8) 6
9) 19
10) −4
11) 9
12) 14
13) 20
14) −21
15) −21
16) 4
17) −16
18) 20
19) 30
20) −9
21) 24
22) −13
23) 45
24) −37
25) 30
26) 4
27) 50
28) 42
29) 33
30) 28
31) 34
32) −16

Multi–Step Equations

1) 1
2) 3
3) 3
4) 7
5) 15
6) 2
7) 9
8) 3
9) 2
10) −3
11) −6
12) −12
13) −4
14) 2
15) −1
16) 16
17) −2
18) −5
19) −6
20) 20
21) −1
22) −2
23) −6
24) 3
25) 3
26) 6
27) 5
28) 13
29) 2
30) 29
31) −3
32) −6

Graphing Single–Variable Inequalities

1)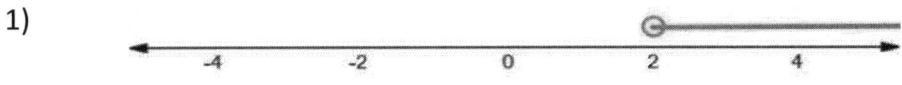

2)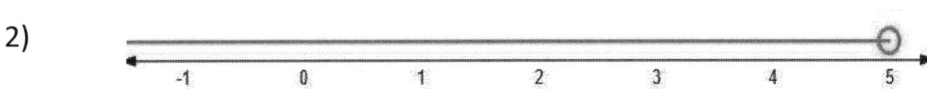

3)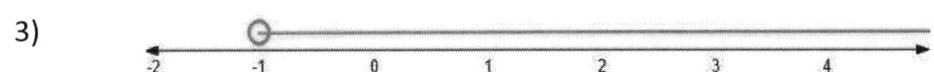

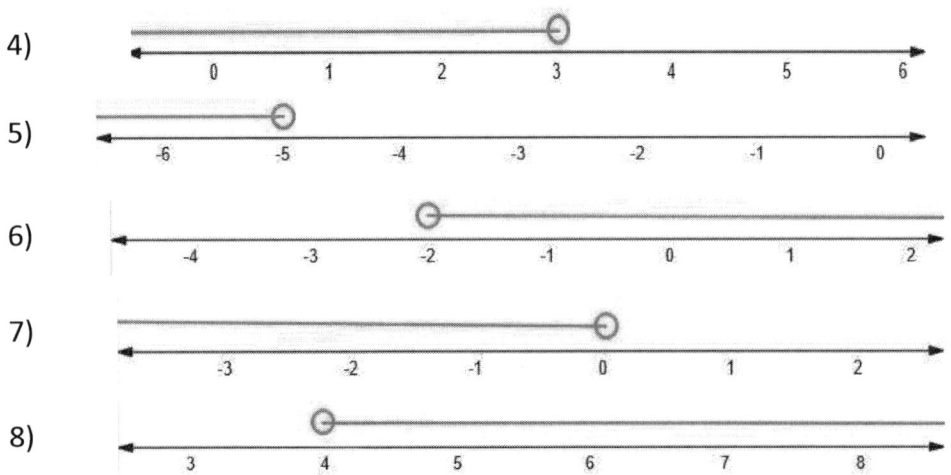

One–Step Inequalities

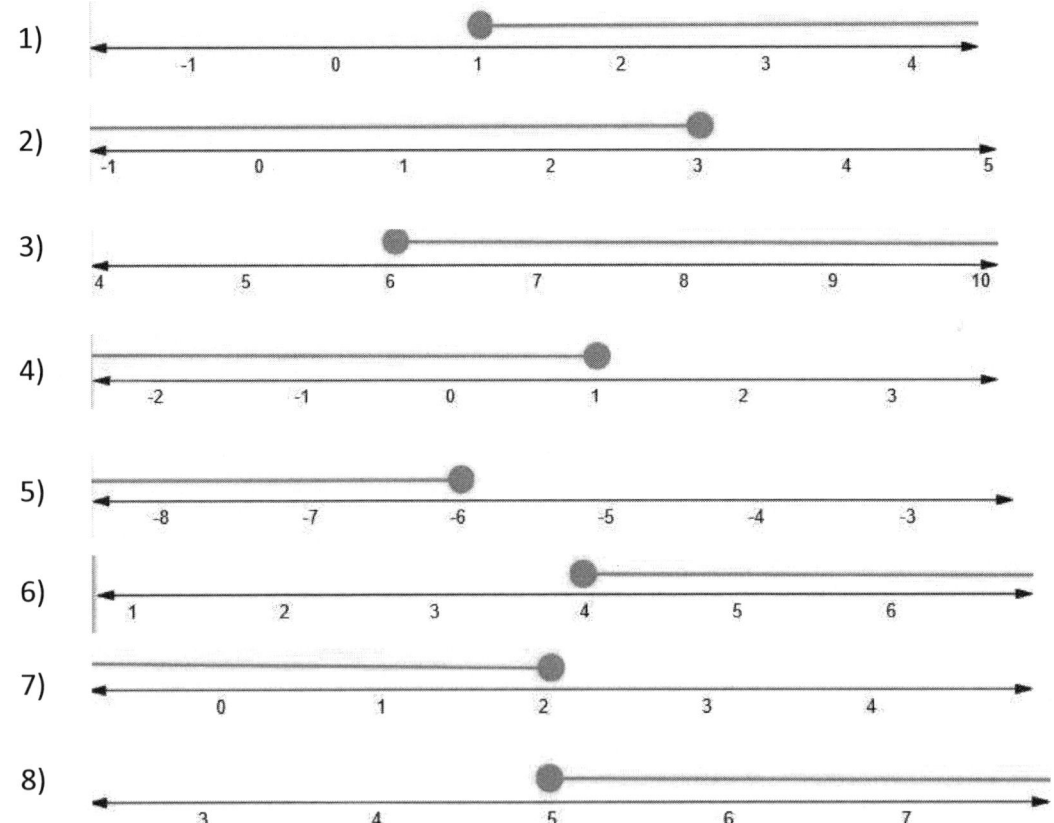

Multi-Step Inequalities

1) $x \leq 8$
2) $x \geq 0$
3) $x \leq 6$
4) $x \geq 7$
5) $x \geq 15$
6) $x \leq 7$
7) $x \leq 2$
8) $x \leq 5$
9) $x \leq 6$

10) $x \leq 2$
11) $x < 10$
12) $x < 12$
13) $x \leq 10$
14) $x < 3$
15) $x \geq 8$
16) $x < 13$

17) $x < 2$
18) $x \leq 4$
19) $x > -4$
20) $x \leq 6$
21) $x < 0$
22) $x \leq 17$
23) $x \leq 4$

24) $x > 5$
25) $x < 9$
26) $x < 7$
27) $x > -2$
28) $x < -15$

Systems of Equations

1) $x = -1, y = 1$
2) $x = 0, y = -3$
3) $x = -4$
4) $x = 1, y = 2$
5) $x = -4, y = -3$
6) $x = 1, y = -2$

7) $x = 1, y = 2$
8) $x = 1, y = 1$
9) $x = 3, y = 2$
10) $x = -4, y = 3$
11) $x = 1, y = 2$
12) $x = 2, y = -6$

13) $x = 0, y = -3$
14) $x = -2, y = -4$
15) $x = 4, y = -2$
16) $x = 5, y = -7$

Systems of Equations Word Problems

1) 14
2) $32
3) 8
4) 5

5) $12
6) 10
7) 34
8) 42, 24

9) 11 $meters$
10) 29

Quadratic Equations

1) $x^2 + 2x - 8$
2) $x^2 + 7x + 6$
3) $x^2 - 2x - 8$
4) $x^2 + 2x - 15$
5) $x^2 - 8x + 12$
6) $2x^2 - 5x - 3$
7) $2x^2 + 7x - 4$
8) $2x^2 + 5x - 12$
9) $3x^2 - 4x - 15$
10) $6x^2 + 2x - 8$

11) $(x - 4)(x - 1)$
12) $(x + 4)(x + 2)$
13) $(x - 3)(x + 4)$
14) $(x - 5)(x - 2)$
15) $(x + 2)(x - 6)$
16) $(2x + 1)(x - 2)$
17) $(2x + 4)(x + 2)$
18) $(3x - 1)(x + 5)$
19) $(3x + 1)(x + 1)$
20) $(2x - 2)(2x - 4)$
21) $x = -2, x = 4$

22) $x = -5, x = -8$
23) $x = -2, x = -3$
24) $x = 3, x = -3$
25) $x = 3, x = 8$
26) $x = -2, x = -5$
27) $x = 4, x = 6$
28) $x = 3, x = -6$
29) $x = 2, x = -1$
30) $x = -2, x = 3$

Chapter 6:

Linear Functions

Topics that you'll practice in this chapter:

- ✓ Finding Slope
- ✓ Graphing Lines Using Line Equation
- ✓ Writing Linear Equations
- ✓ Graphing Linear Inequalities
- ✓ Finding Midpoint
- ✓ Finding Distance of Two Points

"Nature is written in Mathematical language." – *Galileo Galilei*

Finding Slope

✎ **Find the slope of each line.**

1) $y = x - 1$

2) $y = -2x + 5$

3) $y = 2x - 1$

4) $y = -x - 8$

5) $y = 6 + 5x$

6) $y = 2 - 3x$

7) $y = 4x + 12$

8) $y = -6x + 2$

9) $y = -x + 8$

10) $y = 7x - 5$

11) $y = \frac{1}{2}x + 3$

12) $y = -\frac{2}{3}x + 1$

13) $-x + 2y = 5$

14) $2x + 2y = 6$

15) $8y - 2x = 10$

16) $5y - x = 2$

✎ **Find the slope of the line through each pair of points.**

17) $(1, 1), (2, 3)$

18) $(-1, 2), (0, 3)$

19) $(3, -1), (2, 3)$

20) $(-2, -1), (0, 5)$

21) $(5, 1), (2, 4)$

22) $(-3, 1), (-2, 4)$

23) $(6, 2), (7, 4)$

24) $(6, -5), (3, 4)$

25) $(12, -9), (11, -8)$

26) $(7, 4), (5, -2)$

27) $(1, 1), (3, 5)$

28) $(7, -12), (5, 10)$

Graphing Lines Using Line Equation

✎ **Sketch the graph of each line.**

1) $y = 3x - 2$

2) $y = -x + 1$

3) $x + y = 4$

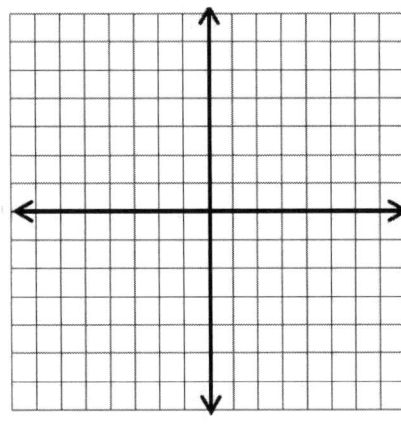
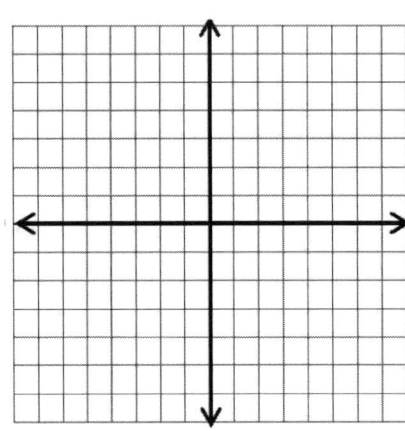
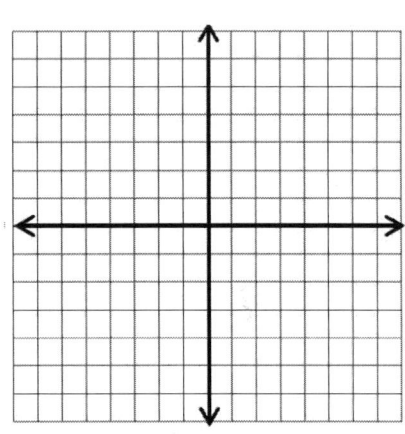

4) $x - y = -5$

5) $2x - y = -4$

6) $3x - 2y = -6$

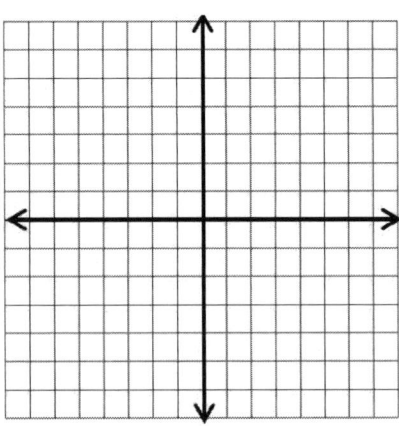
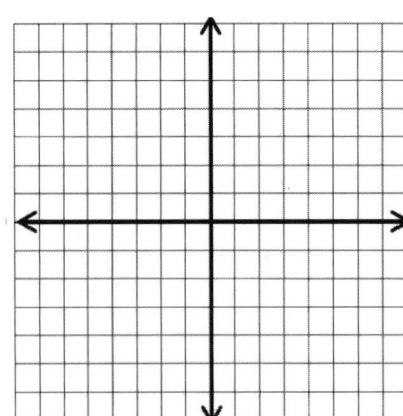
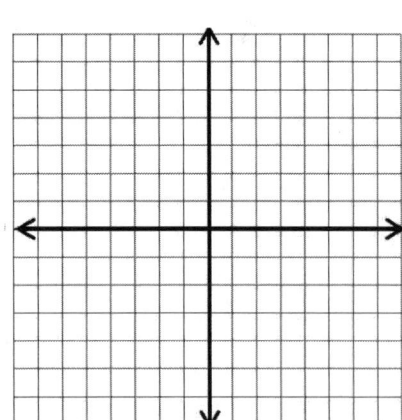

Writing Linear Equations

✎ **Write the equation of the line through the given points.**

1) through: $(1, -2), (2, 3)$

2) through: $(-2, 1), (1, 4)$

3) through: $(-2, 1), (0, 5)$

4) through: $(5, 4), (2, 1)$

5) through: $(-4, 9), (3, 2)$

6) through: $(8, 3), (7, 2)$

7) through: $(7, -2), (5, 2)$

8) through: $(-3, 9), (5, -7)$

9) through: $(6, 8), (4, 14)$

10) through: $(5, 9), (7, -3)$

11) through: $(-2, 8), (-6, -4)$

12) through: $(3, 3), (1, -5)$

13) through: $(8, -5), (-5, 8)$

14) through: $(2, -6), (-1, 3)$

15) through: $(5, 5), (2, -4)$

16) through: $(-1, 8), (2, -7)$

✎ **Solve each problem.**

17) What is the equation of a line with slope 2 and intercept 4? _____

18) What is the equation of a line with slope 4 and intercept 12? _____

19) What is the equation of a line with slope 4 and passes through point $(4, 2)$?
_____

20) What is the equation of a line with slope -2 and passes through point $(-2, 4)$?
_____

21) The slope of a line is -3 and it passes through point $(-1, 5)$. What is the equation of the line? _____

22) The slope of a line is 3 and it passes through point $(-1, 4)$. What is the equation of the line? _____

Graphing Linear Inequalities

✍ **Sketch the graph of each linear inequality.**

1) $y > 3x - 1$

2) $y < -x + 4$

3) $y \leq -5x + 8$

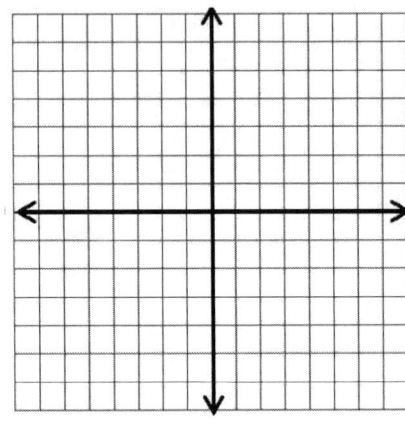
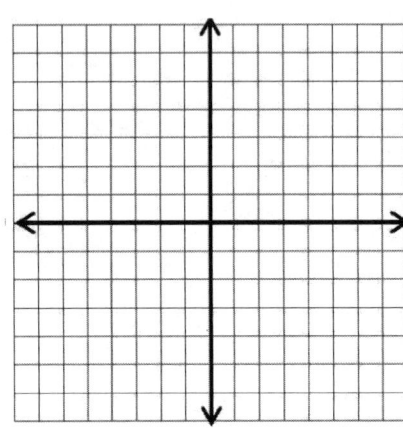
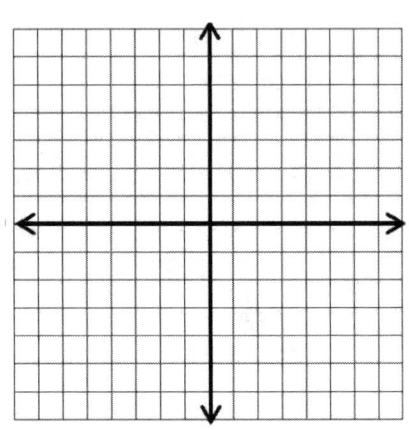

4) $2y \geq 8 + 6x$

5) $y < 2x - 3$

6) $4y \leq -6x + 2$

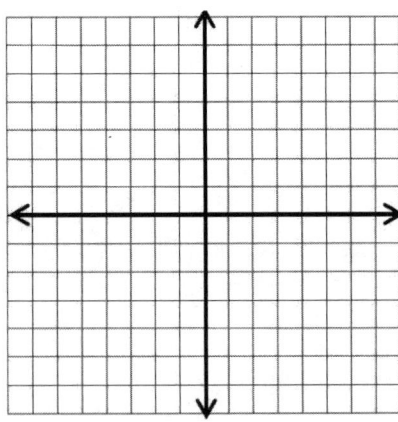
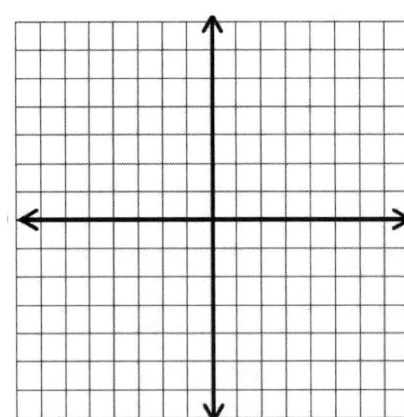
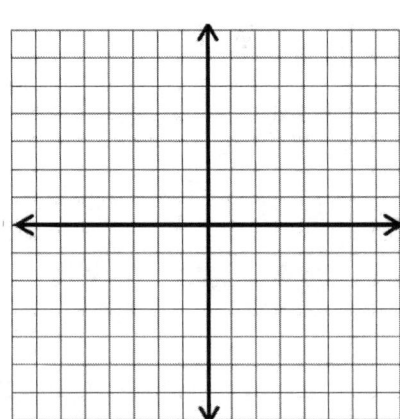

Finding Midpoint

✎ **Find the midpoint of the line segment with the given endpoints.**

1) $(-2, -2), (0, 2)$
2) $(5, 1), (-2, 4)$
3) $(4, -1), (0, 3)$
4) $(-3, 5), (-1, 3)$
5) $(3, -2), (7, -6)$
6) $(-4, -3), (2, -7)$
7) $(5, 0), (-5, 8)$
8) $(-6, 4), (-2, 0)$
9) $(-3, 4), (9, -6)$
10) $(2, 8), (6, -2)$
11) $(4, 7), (-6, 5)$
12) $(9, 3), (-1, -7)$
13) $(-4, 12), (-2, 6)$
14) $(14, 5), (8, -1)$
15) $(11, 7), (-3, 1)$
16) $(-7, -4), (-3, 8)$
17) $(13, 7), (5, 11)$
18) $(-5, -10), (9, -2)$
19) $(8, 15), (-2, 7)$
20) $(13, -2), (5, 10)$
21) $(2, -2), (3, -5)$
22) $(0, 2), (-2, -6)$
23) $(7, 4), (9, -1)$
24) $(4, -5), (0, 8)$

✎ **Solve each problem.**

25) One endpoint of a line segment is $(1, 2)$ and the midpoint of the line segment is $(-1, 4)$. What is the other endpoint? _____

26) One endpoint of a line segment is $(-3, 6)$ and the midpoint of the line segment is $(5, 2)$. What is the other endpoint? _____

27) One endpoint of a line segment is $(-2, -6)$ and the midpoint of the line segment is $(6, 8)$. What is the other endpoint? _____

Finding Distance of Two Points

✎ **Find the distance between each pair of points.**

1) $(2, 1), (-1, -3)$

2) $(-2, -1), (2, 2)$

3) $(-1, 0), (5, 8)$

4) $(-4, -1), (1, 11)$

5) $(3, -2), (-6, -14)$

6) $(-6, 0), (-2, 3)$

7) $(3, 2), (11, 17)$

8) $(-6, -10), (6, -1)$

9) $(5, 9), (-11, -3)$

10) $(9, -3), (3, -11)$

11) $(2, 0), (12, 24)$

12) $(8, 4), (3, -8)$

13) $(4, 2), (-5, -10)$

14) $(-5, 6), (3, 21)$

15) $(0, 8), (-4, 5)$

16) $(-8, -5), (4, 0)$

17) $(3, 5), (-5, -10)$

18) $(-2, 3), (22, 13)$

19) $(7, 2), (-8, -18)$

20) $(-5, 4), (7, 9)$

✎ **Solve each problem.**

21) Triangle ABC is a right triangle on the coordinate system and its vertices are $(-2, 5)$, $(-2, 1)$, and $(1, 1)$. What is the area of triangle ABC? _____

22) Three vertices of a triangle on a coordinate system are $(1, 1)$, $(1, 4)$, and $(5, 4)$. What is the perimeter of the triangle? _____

23) Four vertices of a rectangle on a coordinate system are $(2, 5)$, $(2, 2)$, $(6, 5)$, and $(6, 2)$. What is its perimeter? _____

Answers of Worksheets – Chapter 6

Finding Slope

1) 1
2) -2
3) 2
4) -1
5) 5
6) -3
7) 4
8) -6
9) -1
10) 7

11) $\frac{1}{2}$
12) $-\frac{2}{3}$
13) $\frac{1}{2}$
14) -1
15) $\frac{1}{4}$
16) $\frac{1}{5}$
17) 2
18) 1

19) -4
20) 3
21) -1
22) 3
23) 2
24) -3
25) -1
26) 3
27) 2
28) -11

Graphing Lines Using Line Equation

1) $y = 3x - 2$

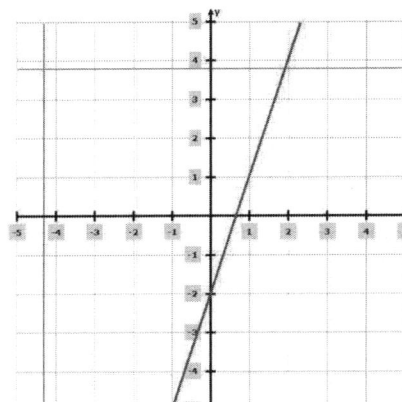

2) $y = -x + 1$

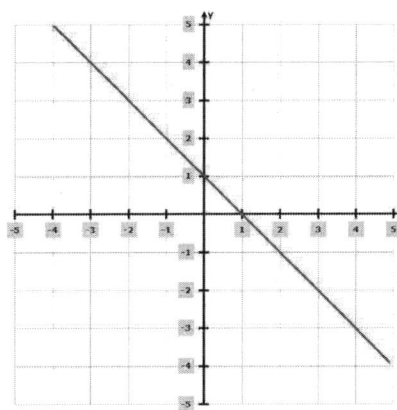

3) $x + y = 4$

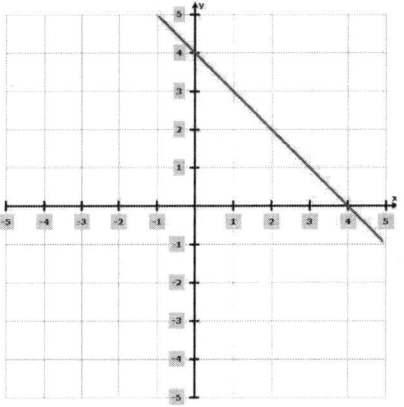

4) $x - y = -5$

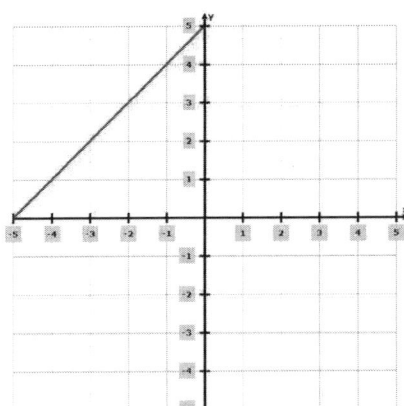

5) $2x - y = -4$

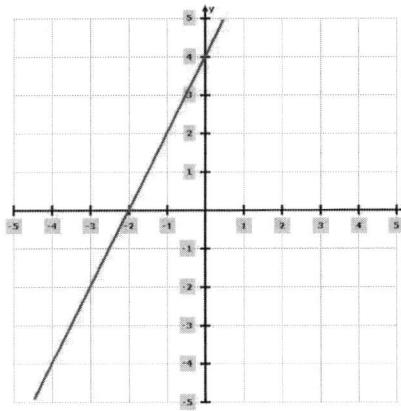

6) $3x - 2y = -6$

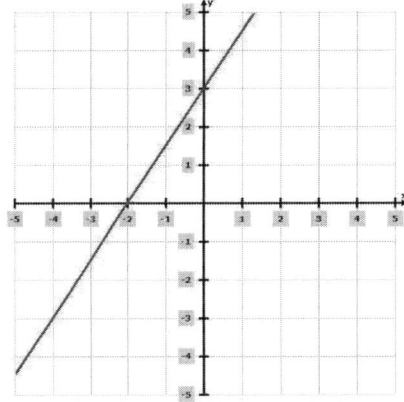

Writing Linear Equations

1) $y = 5x - 7$
2) $y = x + 3$
3) $y = 2x + 5$
4) $y = x - 1$
5) $y = -x + 5$
6) $y = x - 5$
7) $y = -2x + 12$
8) $y = -2x + 3$
9) $y = -3x + 26$
10) $y = -6x + 39$
11) $y = 3x + 14$
12) $y = 4x - 9$
13) $y = -x + 3$
14) $y = -3x$
15) $y = 3x - 10$
16) $y = -5x + 3$
17) $y = 2x + 4$
18) $y = 4x + 12$
19) $y = 4x - 14$
20) $y = -2x + 8$
21) $y = -3x + 2$
22) $y = 3x + 7$

Graphing Linear Inequalities

1) $y > 3x - 1$

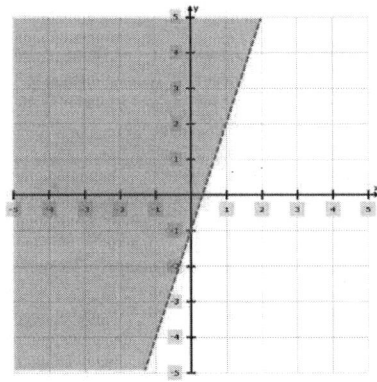

2) $y < -x + 4$

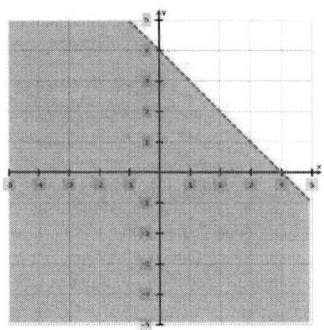

3) $y \leq -5x + 8$

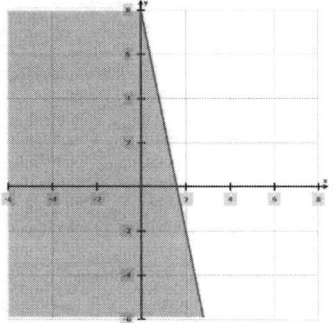

4) $2y \geq 8 + 6x$

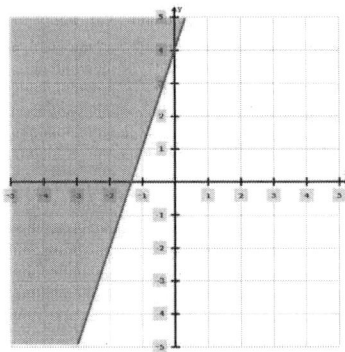

5) $y < 2x - 3$

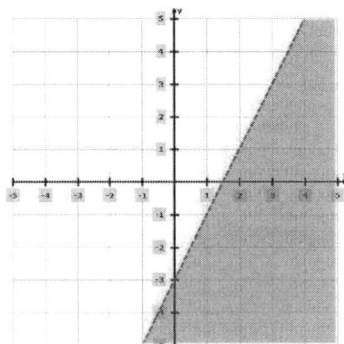

6) $4y \leq -6x + 2$

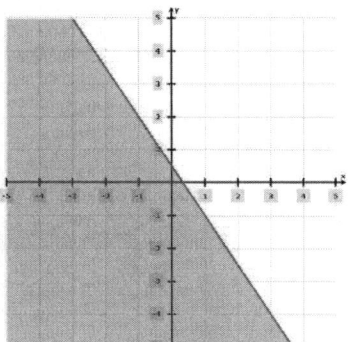

Finding Midpoint

1) $(-1, 0)$
2) $(1.5, 2.5)$
3) $(2, 1)$
4) $(-2, 4)$
5) $(5, -4)$
6) $(-1, -5)$
7) $(0, 4)$
8) $(-4, 2)$
9) $(3, -1)$
10) $(4, 3)$
11) $(-1, 6)$
12) $(4, -2)$
13) $(-3, 9)$
14) $(11, 2)$
15) $(4, 4)$

16) $(-5, 2)$
17) $(9, 9)$
18) $(2, -6)$
19) $(3, 11)$

20) $(9, 4)$
21) $(2.5, -3.5)$
22) $(-1, -2)$
23) $(8, 1.5)$

24) $(2, 1.5)$
25) $(-3, 6)$
26) $(13, -2)$
27) $(14, 22)$

Finding Distance of Two Points

1) 5
2) 5
3) 10
4) 13
5) 15
6) 5
7) 17
8) 15

9) 20
10) 10
11) 26
12) 13
13) 15
14) 17
15) 5
16) 13

17) 17
18) 26
19) 25
20) 13
21) 6 *square units*
22) 12 *units*
23) 14 *units*

Chapter 7:

Exponents

Topics that you'll practice in this chapter:

- ✓ Multiplication Property of Exponents
- ✓ Zero and Negative Exponents
- ✓ Division Property of Exponents
- ✓ Powers of Products and Quotients
- ✓ Negative Exponents and Negative Bases
- ✓ Scientific Notation
- ✓ Square Roots

Mathematics is no more computation than typing is literature.

– John Allen Paulos

Multiplication Property of Exponents

✎ *Simplify and write the answer in exponential form.*

1) $2 \times 2^2 =$

2) $5^3 \times 5 =$

3) $3^2 \times 3^2 =$

4) $4^2 \times 4^2 =$

5) $7^3 \times 7^2 \times 7 =$

6) $2 \times 2^2 \times 2^2 =$

7) $5^3 \times 5^2 \times 5 \times 5 =$

8) $2x \times x =$

9) $x^3 \times x^2 =$

10) $x^4 \times x^4 =$

11) $x^2 \times x^2 \times x^2 =$

12) $6x \times 6x =$

13) $2x^2 \times 2x^2 =$

14) $3x^2 \times x =$

15) $4x^4 \times 4x^4 \times 4x^4 =$

16) $2x^2 \times x^2 =$

17) $x^4 \times 3x =$

18) $x \times 2x^2 =$

19) $5x^4 \times 5x^4 =$

20) $2yx^2 \times 2x =$

21) $3x^4 \times y^2 x^4 =$

22) $y^2 x^3 \times y^5 x^2 =$

23) $4yx^3 \times 2x^2 y^3 =$

24) $6x^2 \times 6x^3 y^4 =$

25) $3x^4 y^5 \times 7x^2 y^3 =$

26) $7x^2 y^5 \times 9xy^3 =$

27) $7xy^4 \times 4x^3 y^3 =$

28) $3x^5 y^3 \times 8x^2 y^3 =$

29) $3x \times y^5 x^3 \times y^4 =$

30) $yx^2 \times 2y^2 x^2 \times 2xy =$

31) $4yx^4 \times 5y^5 x \times xy^3 =$

32) $7x^3 \times 10y^3 x^5 \times 8yx^3 =$

Zero and Negative Exponents

✎ *Evaluate the following expressions.*

1) $1^{-1} =$

2) $2^{-2} =$

3) $0^{15} =$

4) $1^{-10} =$

5) $8^{-1} =$

6) $8^{-2} =$

7) $2^{-4} =$

8) $10^{-2} =$

9) $9^{-1} =$

10) $3^{-2} =$

11) $7^{-2} =$

12) $3^{-4} =$

13) $6^{-2} =$

14) $5^{-3} =$

15) $22^{-1} =$

16) $4^{-2} =$

17) $5^{-2} =$

18) $35^{-1} =$

19) $4^{-3} =$

20) $6^{-3} =$

21) $3^{-5} =$

22) $5^{-2} =$

23) $2^{-3} =$

24) $3^{-3} =$

25) $7^{-3} =$

26) $6^{-3} =$

27) $8^{-3} =$

28) $9^{-2} =$

29) $10^{-3} =$

30) $10^{-9} =$

31) $(\frac{1}{2})^{-1} =$

32) $(\frac{1}{2})^{-2} =$

33) $(\frac{1}{3})^{-2} =$

34) $(\frac{2}{3})^{-2} =$

35) $(\frac{1}{5})^{-3} =$

36) $(\frac{3}{4})^{-2} =$

37) $(\frac{2}{5})^{-2} =$

38) $(\frac{1}{2})^{-8} =$

39) $(\frac{2}{5})^{-3} =$

40) $(\frac{3}{7})^{-2} =$

41) $(\frac{5}{6})^{-3} =$

42) $(\frac{4}{9})^{-2} =$

Division Property of Exponents

✎ *Simplify.*

1) $\dfrac{2^2}{2^3} =$

2) $\dfrac{2^4}{2^2} =$

3) $\dfrac{5^5}{5} =$

4) $\dfrac{3}{3^5} =$

5) $\dfrac{x}{x^3} =$

6) $\dfrac{3 \times 3^3}{3^2 \times 3^4} =$

7) $\dfrac{5^8}{5^3} =$

8) $\dfrac{5 \times 5^6}{5^2 \times 5^7} =$

9) $\dfrac{3^4 \times 3^7}{3^2 \times 3^8} =$

10) $\dfrac{5x}{10x^3} =$

11) $\dfrac{3x^3}{2x^5} =$

12) $\dfrac{12^{\ 3}}{14^{\ 6}} =$

13) $\dfrac{12x^3}{9y^8} =$

14) $\dfrac{25xy^4}{5x^6y^2} =$

15) $\dfrac{2x^4}{7x} =$

16) $\dfrac{16x^2y^8}{4x^3} =$

17) $\dfrac{12x^4}{15^{\ 7}y^9} =$

18) $\dfrac{12yx^4}{10yx^8} =$

19) $\dfrac{16^{\ 4}y}{9x^8y^2} =$

20) $\dfrac{5x^8}{20^{\ 8}} =$

21) $\dfrac{2x^{-5}}{9x^{-2}} =$

Powers of Products and Quotients

✎ **Simplify.**

1) $(4^2)^2 =$

2) $(6^2)^3 =$

3) $(2 \times 2^3)^4 =$

4) $(4 \times 4^4)^2 =$

5) $(3^3 \times 3^2)^3 =$

6) $(5^4 \times 5^5)^2 =$

7) $(2 \times 2^4)^2 =$

8) $(2^6)^2 =$

9) $(11x^5)^2 =$

10) $(4x^2 y^4)^4 =$

11) $(2x^4 y^4)^3 =$

12) $(3x^2 y^2)^2 =$

13) $(3x^4 y^3)^4 =$

14) $(2x^6 y^8)^2 =$

15) $(12x^3 x)^3 =$

16) $(2x^9 x^6)^3 =$

17) $(5x^{10} y^3)^3 =$

18) $(4x^3 x^3)^2 =$

19) $(3x^3 . 5x)^2 =$

20) $(10x^{11} y^3)^2 =$

21) $(9x^7 y^5)^2 =$

22) $(4x^4 y^6)^5 =$

23) $(3x . 4y^3)^2 =$

24) $\left(\dfrac{5x}{x^2}\right)^2 =$

25) $\left(\dfrac{x^4 y^4}{x^2 y^2}\right)^3 =$

26) $\left(\dfrac{25x}{5x^6}\right)^2 =$

27) $\left(\dfrac{x^8}{x^6 y^2}\right)^2 =$

28) $\left(\dfrac{xy^2}{x^3 y^3}\right)^{-2} =$

29) $\left(\dfrac{2xy^4}{x^3}\right)^2 =$

30) $\left(\dfrac{xy^4}{5xy^2}\right)^{-3} =$

Negative Exponents and Negative Bases

✍ **Simplify.**

1) $-6^{-1} =$

2) $-5^{-2} =$

3) $-2^{-4} =$

4) $-x^{-3} =$

5) $2x^{-1} =$

6) $-4x^{-3} =$

7) $-12x^{-5} =$

8) $-5x^{-2}y^{-3} =$

9) $20x^{-4}y^{-1} =$

10) $14a^{-6}b^{-7} =$

11) $-12x^2y^{-3} =$

12) $-\dfrac{25}{x^{-6}} =$

13) $-\dfrac{2x}{a^{-4}} =$

14) $\left(-\dfrac{1}{3}\right)^{-2} =$

15) $\left(-\dfrac{3}{4}\right)^{-2} =$

16) $-\dfrac{9}{a^{-7}b^{-2}} =$

17) $-\dfrac{5x}{x^{-3}} =$

18) $-\dfrac{a^{-3}}{b^{-2}} =$

19) $-\dfrac{5}{x^{-3}} =$

20) $\dfrac{7b}{-9c^{-4}} =$

21) $\dfrac{7ab}{a^{-3}b^{-1}} =$

22) $-\dfrac{5n^{-2}}{10p^{-3}} =$

23) $\dfrac{4a^{-2}}{-3c^{-2}} =$

24) $\left(\dfrac{3a}{2c}\right)^{-2} =$

25) $\left(-\dfrac{5x}{3y}\right)^{-3} =$

26) $\dfrac{4ab^{-2}}{-3c^{-2}} =$

27) $\left(-\dfrac{x^3}{x^4}\right)^{-2} =$

28) $\left(-\dfrac{x^{-2}}{3x^2}\right)^{-3} =$

29) $\left(-\dfrac{x^{-4}}{x^2}\right)^{-2} =$

Scientific Notation

✎ **Write each number in scientific notation.**

1) $0.113 =$

2) $0.02 =$

3) $2.5 =$

4) $20 =$

5) $60 =$

6) $0.004 =$

7) $78 =$

8) $1,600 =$

9) $1,450 =$

10) $91,000 =$

11) $2,000,000 =$

12) $0.0000006 =$

13) $354,000 =$

14) $0.000325 =$

15) $0.00023 =$

16) $56,000,000 =$

17) $21,000 =$

18) $78,000,000 =$

19) $0.0000022 =$

20) $0.00012 =$

✎ **Write each number in standard notation.**

21) $3 \times 10^{-1} =$

22) $5 \times 10^{-2} =$

23) $1.2 \times 10^{3} =$

24) $2 \times 10^{-4} =$

25) $1.5 \times 10^{-2} =$

26) $4 \times 10^{3} =$

27) $9 \times 10^{5} =$

28) $1.12 \times 10^{4} =$

29) $3 \times 10^{-5} =$

30) $8.3 \times 10^{-5} =$

Answers of Worksheets – Chapter 7

Multiplication Property of Exponents

1) 2^3
2) 5^4
3) 3^4
4) 4^4
5) 7^6
6) 2^5
7) 5^7
8) $2x^2$
9) x^5
10) x^8
11) x^6
12) $36x^2$
13) $4x^4$
14) $3x^3$
15) $64x^{12}$
16) $2x^4$
17) $3x^5$
18) $2x^3$
19) $25x^8$
20) $4x^3y$
21) $3x^8y^2$
22) x^5y^7
23) $8x^5y^4$
24) $36x^5y^4$
25) $21x^6y^8$
26) $63x^3y^8$
27) $28x^4y^7$
28) $24x^7y^6$
29) $3x^4y^9$
30) $4x^5y^4$
31) $20x^6y^9$
32) $560x^{11}y^4$

Zero and Negative Exponents

1) 1
2) $\frac{1}{4}$
3) 0
4) 1
5) $\frac{1}{8}$
6) $\frac{1}{64}$
7) $\frac{1}{16}$
8) $\frac{1}{100}$
9) $\frac{1}{9}$
10) $\frac{1}{9}$
11) $\frac{1}{49}$
12) $\frac{1}{81}$
13) $\frac{1}{36}$
14) $\frac{1}{125}$
15) $\frac{1}{22}$
16) $\frac{1}{16}$
17) $\frac{1}{25}$
18) $\frac{1}{35}$
19) $\frac{1}{64}$
20) $\frac{1}{216}$
21) $\frac{1}{243}$
22) $\frac{1}{25}$
23) $\frac{1}{8}$
24) $\frac{1}{27}$
25) $\frac{1}{343}$
26) $\frac{1}{216}$
27) $\frac{1}{512}$
28) $\frac{1}{81}$
29) $\frac{1}{1,000}$
30) $\frac{1}{1,000,000,000}$
31) 2
32) 4
33) 9
34) $\frac{9}{4}$
35) 125
36) $\frac{16}{9}$
37) $\frac{25}{4}$
38) 256
39) $\frac{125}{8}$
40) $\frac{49}{9}$
41) $\frac{216}{125}$
42) $\frac{81}{16}$

Division Property of Exponents

1) $\frac{1}{2}$
2) 2^2
3) 5^4
4) $\frac{1}{3^4}$
5) $\frac{1}{x^2}$
6) $\frac{1}{3^2}$
7) 5^5
8) 1
9) 3
10) $\frac{1}{2x^2}$
11) $\frac{3}{2x^2}$
12) $\frac{6}{7x^3}$
13) $\frac{4x^3}{3y^8}$
14) $\frac{5y^2}{x^5}$
15) $\frac{2x^3}{7}$
16) $\frac{4y^8}{x}$
17) $\frac{4}{5x^3y^9}$
18) $\frac{6}{5x^4}$
19) $\frac{16}{9x^4y}$
20) $\frac{1}{4}$
21) $\frac{2}{9x^3}$

Powers of Products and Quotients

1) 4^4
2) 6^6
3) 2^{16}
4) 4^{10}
5) 3^{15}
6) 5^{18}
7) 2^{10}
8) 2^{12}
9) $121x^{10}$
10) $256x^8y^{16}$
11) $8x^{12}y^{12}$
12) $9x^4y^4$
13) $81x^{16}y^{12}$
14) $4x^{12}y^{16}$
15) $1{,}728x^{12}$
16) $8x^{45}$
17) $125x^{30}y^9$
18) $16x^{12}$
19) $225x^8$
20) $100x^{22}y^6$
21) $81x^{14}y^{10}$
22) $1{,}024x^{20}y^{30}$
23) $144x^2y^6$
24) $\frac{25}{x^2}$
25) x^2y^2
26) $\frac{25y^4}{x^{10}}$
27) $\frac{x^4}{y^4}$
28) x^4y^2
29) $\frac{4y^8}{x^4}$
30) $\frac{125}{y^6}$

Negative Exponents and Negative Bases

1) $-\frac{1}{6}$
2) $-\frac{1}{25}$
3) $-\frac{1}{16}$
4) $-\frac{1}{x^3}$
5) $\frac{2}{x}$
6) $-\frac{4}{x^3}$
7) $-\frac{12}{x^5}$
8) $-\frac{5}{x^5y^3}$
9) $\frac{20}{x^4y}$
10) $\frac{14}{a^6b^7}$
11) $-\frac{12x^2}{y^3}$
12) $-25x^6$
13) $-2xa^4$
14) 9
15) $\frac{16}{9}$
16) $-9a^7b^2$
17) $-5x^4$

18) $-\dfrac{b^2}{a^3}$

19) $-5x^3$

20) $-\dfrac{7bc^4}{9}$

21) $7a^4b^2$

22) $-\dfrac{p^3}{2n^2}$

23) $-\dfrac{4ac^2}{3b^2}$

24) $\dfrac{4c^2}{9a^2}$

25) $-\dfrac{27\ ^3z^3}{125x^3}$

26) $-\dfrac{4a\ ^2}{3b^2}$

27) x^2

28) $-81x^{12}$

29) x^{12}

Writing Scientific Notation

1) 1.13×10^{-1}
2) 2×10^{-2}
3) 2.5×10^0
4) 2×10^1
5) 6×10^1
6) 4×10^{-3}
7) 7.8×10^1
8) 1.6×10^3
9) 1.45×10^3
10) 9.1×10^4
11) 2×10^6
12) 6×10^{-7}
13) 3.54×10^5
14) 3.25×10^{-4}
15) 2.3×10^{-4}
16) 5.6×10^7
17) 2.1×10^4
18) 7.8×10^7
19) 2.2×10^{-6}
20) 1.2×10^{-4}
21) 0.3
22) 0.05
23) 1,200
24) 0.0002
25) 0.015
26) 4,000
27) 900,000
28) 11,200
29) 0.00003
30) 0.000083

Chapter 8:

Polynomials

Topics that you'll practice in this chapter:

✓ Writing Polynomials in Standard Form

✓ Simplifying Polynomials

✓ Adding and Subtracting Polynomials

✓ Multiplying Monomials

✓ Multiplying and Dividing Monomials

✓ Multiplying a Polynomial and a Monomial

✓ Multiplying Binomials

✓ Factoring Trinomials

✓ Operations with Polynomials

Mathematics is the supreme judge; from its decisions there is no appeal.– Tobias Dantzig

Writing Polynomials in Standard Form

✎ *Write each polynomial in standard form.*

1) $9x - 7x =$

2) $-3 + 16x - 16x =$

3) $3x^2 - 5x^3 =$

4) $3 + 4x^3 - 3 =$

5) $2x^2 + 1x - 6x^3 =$

6) $-x^2 + 2x^3 =$

7) $2x + 4x^3 - 2x^2 =$

8) $-2x^2 + 4x - 6x^3 =$

9) $2x^2 + 2 - 5x =$

10) $12 - 7x + 9x^4 =$

11) $5x^2 + 13x - 2x^3 =$

12) $10 + 6x^2 - x^3 =$

13) $12x^2 - 7x + 9x^3 =$

14) $5x^4 - 3x^2 - 2x^3 =$

15) $-12 + 3x^2 - 6x^4 =$

16) $5x^2 - 9x^5 + 8x^3 - 11 =$

17) $4x^2 - 2x^5 + 14 - 7x^4 =$

18) $-x^2 + 2x - 5x^3 - 4x =$

19) $8x^5 + 11x^3 - 6x^5 - 8x^2 =$

20) $5x^2 - 12x^4 + 4x^2 + 5x^3 =$

21) $7x^3 - 6x^4 - 3x^2 + 22x^3 =$

22) $9x^2 + x^4 + 12x^3 - 5x^4 =$

23) $3x(2x + 5 - 2x^2) =$

24) $11x(x^5 + 2x^3) =$

25) $5x(3x^2 + 2x + 1) =$

26) $7x(3 - x + 6x^3) =$

27) $2x(3x^2 - 4x^4 + 3) =$

28) $6x(4x^5 + 7x^3 - 2) =$

29) $5x(3x^2 + 2x^3 + x) =$

30) $7x(3x - x^2 + 6x^4) =$

Simplifying Polynomials

✍ Simplify each expression.

1) $5(2x - 10) =$

2) $2x(4x - 2) =$

3) $4x(5x - 3) =$

4) $3x(7x + 3) =$

5) $4x(8x - 4) =$

6) $5x(5x + 4) =$

7) $(2x - 3)(x - 4) =$

8) $(x - 5)(3x + 4) =$

9) $(x - 5)(x - 3) =$

10) $(3x + 8)(3x - 8) =$

11) $(3x - 8)(3x - 4) =$

12) $3x^2 + 3x^2 - 2x^3 =$

13) $2x - x^2 + 6x^3 + 4 =$

14) $5x + 2x^2 - 9x^3 =$

15) $7x^2 + 5x^4 - 2x^3 =$

16) $-3x^2 + 5x^3 + 6x^4 =$

17) $-8x^2 + 2x^3 - 10x^4 + 5x =$

18) $11 - 6x^2 + 5x^2 - 12x^3 + 22 =$

19) $2x^2 - 2x + 3x^3 + 12x - 22x =$

20) $11 - 4x^2 + 3x^2 - 7x^3 + 3 =$

21) $2x^5 - x^3 + 8x^2 - 2x^5 =$

22) $(2x^3 - 1) + (3x^3 - 2x^3) =$

23) $3(4x^4 - 4x^3 - 5x^4) =$

24) $-5(x^6 + 10) - 8(14 - x^6) =$

25) $3x^2 - 5x^3 - x + 10 - 2x^2 =$

26) $11 - 3x^2 + 2x^2 - 5x^3 + 7 =$

27) $(8x^2 - 3x) - (5x - 5 - 8x^2) =$

28) $3x^2 - 5x^3 - x(2x^2 + 4x) =$

29) $4x + 8x^3 - 4 - 3(x^3 - 2) =$

30) $12 + 2x^2 - (8x^3 - x^2 + 6x^3) =$

31) $-2(x^4 + 6) - 5(10 + x^4) =$

32) $(8x^3 - 2x) - (5x - 2x^3) =$

Adding and Subtracting Polynomials

✎ **Add or subtract expressions.**

1) $(-x^2 - 2) + (2x^2 + 1) =$

2) $(2x^2 + 3) - (3 - 4x^2) =$

3) $(2x^3 + 3x^2) - (x^3 + 8) =$

4) $(4x^3 - x^2) + (3x^2 - 5x) =$

5) $(7x^3 + 9x) - (3x^3 + 2) =$

6) $(2x^3 - 2) + (2x^3 + 2) =$

7) $(4x^3 + 5) - (7 - 2x^3) =$

8) $(4x^2 + 2x^3) - (2x^3 + 5) =$

9) $(4x^2 - x) + (3x - 5x^2) =$

10) $(7x + 9) - (3x + 9) =$

11) $(4x^4 - 2x) - (6x - 2x^4) =$

12) $(12x - 4x^3) - (8x^3 + 6x) =$

13) $(2x^3 - 8x^2) - (5x^2 - 3x) =$

14) $(2x^2 - 6) + (9x^2 - 4x^3) =$

15) $(4x^3 + 3x^4) - (x^4 - 5x^3) =$

16) $(-2x^3 - 2x) + (6x - 2x^3) =$

17) $(2x - 4x^4) - (8x^4 + 3x) =$

18) $(2x - 8x^2) - (5x^4 - 3x^2) =$

19) $(2x^3 - 6) + (9x^3 - 4x^2) =$

20) $(4x^3 + 3x^4) - (x^4 - 5x^3) =$

21) $(-2x^2 + 10x^4 + x^3) + (4x^3 + 3x^4 + 8x^2) =$

22) $(3x^2 - 6x^5 - 2x) - (-2x^2 - 6x^5 + 2x) =$

23) $(5x + 9x^3 - 3x^5) + (8x^3 + 3x^5 - 2x) =$

24) $(3x^5 - 2x^4 - 4x) - (4x^2 + 10x^4 - 3x) =$

25) $(13x^2 - 6x^5 - 2x) - (-10x^2 - 11x^5 + 9x) =$

26) $(-12x^4 + 10x^5 + 2x^3) + (14x^3 + 23x^5 + 8x^4) =$

Multiplying Monomials

✎ **Simplify each expression.**

1) $4u^9 \times (-2u^3) =$

2) $(-2p^7) \times (-3p^2) =$

3) $3xy^2z^3 \times 2z^2 =$

4) $5u^5t \times 3ut^2 =$

5) $(-9a^6) \times (-5a^2b^4) =$

6) $-2a^3b^2 \times 4a^2b =$

7) $2xy^2 \times x^2y^3 =$

8) $3p^2q^4 \times (-2pq^3) =$

9) $4s^5t^2 \times 4st^3 =$

10) $(-6x^3y^2) \times 3x^2y =$

11) $2xy^2z \times 4z^2 =$

12) $4xy \times x^2y =$

13) $4pq^3 \times (-2p^4q) =$

14) $8s^4t^2 \times st^5 =$

15) $12p^3 \times (-3p^4) =$

16) $(-4p^2q^3r) \times 6pq^2r^3 =$

17) $(-8a^4) \times -12a^6b) =$

18) $3u^4v^2 \times (-7u^2v^3) =$

19) $4u^3 \times (-2u) =$

20) $-6xy^2 \times 3x^2y =$

21) $12y^2z^3 \times (-y^2z) =$

22) $5a^2bc^2 \times 2abc^2 =$

23) $(-7p^3q^5) \times (-4p^2q^3) =$

24) $4u^5v^2 \times (-8u^3v^2) =$

25) $12y^3z^4 \times (-y^6z) =$

26) $(-4pq^5r^3) \times 6p^2q^4r =$

27) $5ab^4c^2 \times 2a^5bc^2 =$

28) $2x^4yz^3 \times 3x^2y^4z^2 =$

Multiplying and Dividing Monomials

✎ *Simplify each expression.*

1) $(2x^2)(x^3) =$

2) $(3x^4)(2x^4) =$

3) $(6x^5)(2x^2) =$

4) $(4x^3)(3x^5) =$

5) $(15x^4)(3x^9) =$

6) $(2yx^2)(3y^2x^3) =$

7) $(2x^2y)(x^2y^3) =$

8) $(-2x^3y^4)(3x^3y^2) =$

9) $(-5x^3y^2)(-2x^4y^5) =$

10) $(9x^5y)(-3x^3y^3) =$

11) $(8x^7y^2)(6x^5y^4) =$

12) $(7x^4y^6)(4x^3y^4) =$

13) $(12x^2y^9)(7x^9y^{12}) =$

14) $(6x^2y^5)(5x^3y^2) =$

15) $(9x^2y^9)(4x^{10}y^9) =$

16) $(-10x^4y^8)(2x^9y^5) =$

17) $\dfrac{4x^2y^3}{xy^2} =$

18) $\dfrac{2x^4y^3}{2x^3y} =$

19) $\dfrac{8x^2y^2}{4x} =$

20) $\dfrac{6x^3y^4}{2x^2y^3} =$

21) $\dfrac{12x^6y^8}{4x^4y^2} =$

22) $\dfrac{26x^9y^5}{2x^3y^4} =$

23) $\dfrac{80\ ^{12}y^9}{10\ ^6y^7} =$

24) $\dfrac{95\ ^{18}y^7}{5x^9y^2} =$

25) $\dfrac{200x^3y^8}{40x^3y^7} =$

26) $\dfrac{-15x^{17}y^{13}}{3x^6y^9} =$

27) $\dfrac{-64x^8y^{10}}{8x^3y^7} =$

Multiplying a Polynomial and a Monomial

✎ **Find each product.**

1) $x(x + 3) =$

2) $8(2 - x) =$

3) $2x(2x + 1) =$

4) $x(-x + 3) =$

5) $3x(3x - 2) =$

6) $5(3x - 6y) =$

7) $8x(7x - 4) =$

8) $3x(9x + 2y) =$

9) $6x(x + 2y) =$

10) $9x(2x + 4y) =$

11) $12x(3x + 9) =$

12) $11x(2x - 11y) =$

13) $2x(6x - 6y) =$

14) $2x(3x - 6y + 3) =$

15) $5x(3x^2 + 2y^2) =$

16) $13x(4x + 8y) =$

17) $5(2x^2 - 9y^2) =$

18) $3x(-2x^2y + 3y) =$

19) $-2(2x^2 - 2xy + 2) =$

20) $3(x^2 - 4xy - 8) =$

21) $2x(2x^2 - 3xy + 2x) =$

22) $-x(-x^2 - 5x + 4xy) =$

23) $9(x^2 + xy - 8y^2) =$

24) $3x(2x^2 - 3x + 8) =$

25) $20(2x^2 - 8x - 5) =$

26) $x^2(-x^2 + 3x + 7) =$

27) $x^3(x^2 + 12 - 2x) =$

28) $6x^3(3x^2 - 2x + 2) =$

29) $8x^2(3x^2 - 5xy + 7y^2) =$

30) $2x^2(3x^2 - 5x + 12) =$

31) $2x^3(2x^2 + 5x - 4) =$

32) $5x(6x^2 - 5xy + 2y^2) =$

Multiplying Binomials

✏️ *Find each product.*

1) $(x + 2)(x + 2) =$

2) $(x - 3)(x + 2) =$

3) $(x - 2)(x - 4) =$

4) $(x + 3)(x + 2) =$

5) $(x - 4)(x - 5) =$

6) $(x + 5)(x + 2) =$

7) $(x - 6)(x + 3) =$

8) $(x - 8)(x - 4) =$

9) $(x + 2)(x + 8) =$

10) $(x - 2)(x + 4) =$

11) $(x + 4)(x + 4) =$

12) $(x + 5)(x + 5) =$

13) $(x - 3)(x + 3) =$

14) $(x - 2)(x + 2) =$

15) $(x + 3)(x + 3) =$

16) $(x + 4)(x + 6) =$

17) $(x - 7)(x + 7) =$

18) $(x - 7)(x + 2) =$

19) $(2x + 2)(x + 3) =$

20) $(2x - 3)(2x + 4) =$

21) $(x - 8)(2x + 8) =$

22) $(x - 7)(x - 6) =$

23) $(x - 8)(x + 8) =$

24) $(3x - 2)(4x + 2) =$

25) $(2x - 5)(x + 7) =$

26) $(5x - 4)(3x + 3) =$

27) $(6x + 9)(4x + 9) =$

28) $(2x - 6)(5x + 6) =$

29) $(x + 4)(4x - 8) =$

30) $(6x - 4)(6x + 4) =$

31) $(3x + 3)(3x - 4) =$

32) $(x^2 + 2)(x^2 - 2) =$

Factoring Trinomials

✎ **Factor each trinomial.**

1) $x^2 + 8x + 15 =$

2) $x^2 - 5x + 6 =$

3) $x^2 + 6x + 8 =$

4) $x^2 - 6x + 8 =$

5) $x^2 - 8x + 16 =$

6) $x^2 - 7x + 12 =$

7) $x^2 + 11x + 18 =$

8) $x^2 + 2x - 24 =$

9) $x^2 + 4x - 12 =$

10) $x^2 - 10x + 9 =$

11) $x^2 + 5x - 14 =$

12) $x^2 - 6x - 27 =$

13) $x^2 - 11x - 42 =$

14) $x^2 + 22x + 121 =$

15) $6x^2 + x - 12 =$

16) $x^2 - 17x + 30 =$

17) $3x^2 + 11x - 4 =$

18) $10x^2 + 33x - 7 =$

19) $x^2 + 24x + 144 =$

20) $8x^2 + 10x - 3 =$

✎ **Solve each problem.**

21) The area of a rectangle is $x^2 + 2x - 24$. If the width of rectangle is $x - 4$, what is its length? _____

22) The area of a parallelogram is $8x^2 + 2x - 6$ and its height is $2x + 2$. What is the base of the parallelogram? _____

23) The area of a rectangle is $18x^2 + 9x - 2$. If the width of the rectangle is $6x - 1$, what is its length? _____

Operations with Polynomials

✎ *Find each product.*

1) $9(6x + 2) =$ _____

2) $8(3x + 7) =$ _____

3) $5(6x - 1) =$ _____

4) $-3(8x - 3) =$ _____

5) $3x^2(6x - 5) =$ _____

6) $5x^2(7x - 2) =$ _____

7) $6x^3(-3x + 4) =$ _____

8) $-7x^4(2x - 4) =$ _____

9) $8(x^2 + 2x - 3) =$ _____

10) $4(4x^2 - 2x + 1) =$ _____

11) $2(3x^2 + 2x - 2) =$ _____

12) $8x(5x^2 + 3x + 8) =$ _____

13) $(9x + 1)(3x - 1) =$ _____

14) $(4x + 5)(6x - 5) =$ _____

15) $(7x + 3)(5x - 6) =$ _____

16) $(3x - 4)(3x + 8) =$ _____

✎ *Solve each problem.*

17) The measures of two sides of a triangle are $(2x + 3y)$ and $(5x - 2y)$. If the perimeter of the triangle is $(12x + 5y)$, what is the measure of the third side? _____

18) The height of a triangle is $(4x + 5)$ and its base is $(2x - 2)$. What is the area of the triangle? _____

19) One side of a square is $(6x + 9)$. What is the area of the square? _____

20) The length of a rectangle is $(5x - 2y)$ and its width is $(12x + 2y)$. What is the perimeter of the rectangle? _____

21) The side of a cube measures $(x + 2)$. What is the volume of the cube? _____

22) If the perimeter of a rectangle is $(16x + 8y)$ and its width is $(2x + y)$, what is the length of the rectangle? _____

Answers of Worksheets – Chapter 8

Writing Polynomials in Standard Form

1) $2x$
2) -3
3) $-5x^3 + 3x^3$
4) $4x^3$
5) $-6x^3 + 2x^3 + x$
6) $2x^3 - x^2$
7) $4x^3 - 2x^2 + 2x$
8) $-6x^3 - 2x^2 + 4x$
9) $2x^2 - 5x + 2$
10) $9x^4 - 7x + 12$
11) $-2x^3 + 5x^2 + 13x$
12) $-x^3 + 6x^2 + 10$
13) $9x^3 + 12x^2 - 7x$
14) $5x^4 - 2x^3 - 3x^2$
15) $-6x^4 + 3x^2 - 12$
16) $-9x^5 + 8x^3 + 5x^2 - 11$

17) $-2x^5 - 7x^4 + 4x^2 + 14$
18) $-5x^3 - x^2 - 2x$
19) $2x^5 + 11x^3 - 8x^2$
20) $-12x^4 + 5x^3 + 9x^2$
21) $-6x^4 + 29x^3 - 3x^2$
22) $-4x^4 + 12x^3 + 9x^2$
23) $-6x^3 + 6x^2 + 15x$
24) $11x^6 + 22x^4$
25) $15x^3 + 10x^2 + 5x$
26) $42x^4 - 7x^2 + 21x$
27) $-8x^5 + 6x^3 + 6x$
28) $24x^6 + 42x^4 - 12x$
29) $10x^4 + 15x^3 + 5x^2$
30) $42x^5 - 7x^3 + 21x^2$

Simplifying Polynomials

1) $10x - 50$
2) $8x^2 - 4x$
3) $20x^2 - 12x$
4) $21x^2 + 9x$
5) $32x^2 - 16x$
6) $25x^2 + 20x$
7) $2x^2 - 11x + 12$
8) $3x^2 - 11x - 20$
9) $x^2 - 8x + 15$
10) $9x^2 - 64$
11) $9x^2 - 36x + 32$
12) $-2x^3 + 6x^2$
13) $6x^3 - x^2 + 2x + 4$
14) $-9x^3 + 2x^2 + 5x$
15) $5x^4 - 2x^3 + 7x^2$
16) $6x^4 + 5x^3 - 3x^2$

17) $-10x^4 + 2x^3 - 8x^2 + 5x$
18) $-12x^3 - x^2 + 33$
19) $3x^3 + 2x^2 - 12x$
20) $-7x^3 - x^2 + 14$
21) $-x^3 + 8x^2$
22) $3x^3 - 1$
23) $-3x^4 - 12x^3$
24) $3x^6 - 162$
25) $-5x^3 + x^2 - x + 10$
26) $-5x^3 - x^2 + 18$
27) $16x^2 - 8x + 5$
28) $-5x^3 - x^2$
29) $5x^3 + 4x + 2$
30) $-14x^3 + 3x^2 + 12$
31) $-7x^4 - 62$
32) $10x^3 - 7x$

Adding and Subtracting Polynomials

1) $x^2 - 1$
2) $6x^2$
3) $x^3 + 3x^2 - 8$
4) $4x^3 + 2x^2 - 5x$
5) $4x^3 + 9x - 2$
6) $4x^3$
7) $6x^3 - 2$
8) $4x^2 - 5$
9) $-x^2 + 2x$
10) $4x$
11) $6x^4 - 8x$
12) $-12x^3 + 6x$
13) $2x^3 - 13x^2 + 3x$
14) $-4x^3 + 11x^2 - 6$
15) $2x^4 + 9x^3$
16) $-4x^3 + 4x$
17) $-12x^4 - x$
18) $-5x^4 - 5x^2 + 2x$
19) $11x^3 - 4x^2 - 6$
20) $2x^4 + 9x^3$
21) $13x^4 + 5x^3 + 6x^2$
22) $5x^2 - 4x$
23) $17x^3 + 3x$
24) $3x^5 - 12x^4 - 4x^2 - x$
25) $5x^5 + 23x^2 - 11x$
26) $33x^5 - 4x^4 + 16x^3$

Multiplying Monomials

1) $-8u^{12}$
2) $6p^9$
3) $6xy^2z^5$
4) $15u^6t^3$
5) $45a^8b^4$
6) $-8a^5b^3$
7) $2x^3y^5$
8) $-6p^3q^7$
9) $16s^6t^5$
10) $-18x^5y^3$
11) $8xy^2z^3$
12) $4x^3y^2$
13) $-8p^5q^4$
14) $8s^5t^7$
15) $-36p^7$
16) $-24p^3q^4r^4$
17) $96a^{10}b$
18) $-21u^6v^5$
19) $-8u^4$
20) $-18x^3y^3$
21) $-12y^4z^4$
22) $10a^3b^2c^4$
23) $28p^5q^8$
24) $-32u^8v^4$
25) $-12y^9z^5$
26) $-24p^3q^9r^4$
27) $10a^6b^5c^4$
28) $6x^6y^5z^5$

Multiplying and Dividing Monomials

1) $2x^5$
2) $6x^8$
3) $12x^7$
4) $12x^8$
5) $45x^{13}$
6) $6x^5y^3$
7) $2x^4y^4$
8) $-6x^6y^6$
9) $10x^7y^7$
10) $-27x^8y^4$
11) $48x^{12}y^6$
12) $28x^7y^{10}$
13) $84x^{11}y^{21}$
14) $30x^5y^7$
15) $36x^{12}y^{18}$
16) $-20x^{13}y^{13}$
17) $4xy$
18) xy^2
19) $2xy$
20) $3xy$
21) $3x^2y^6$
22) $13x^6y$
23) $8x^6y^2$
24) $19x^9y^5$

25) $5y$ 26) $-5x^{11}y^4$ 27) $-8x^5y^3$

Multiplying a Polynomial and a Monomial

1) $x^2 + 3x$
2) $-8x + 16$
3) $4x^2 + 2x$
4) $-x^2 + 3x$
5) $9x^2 - 6x$
6) $15x - 30y$
7) $56x^2 - 32x$
8) $27x^2 + 6xy$
9) $6x^2 + 12xy$
10) $18x^2 + 36xy$
11) $36x^2 + 108x$
12) $22x^2 - 121xy$
13) $12x^2 - 12xy$
14) $6x^2 - 12xy + 6x$
15) $15x^3 + 10xy^2$
16) $52x^2 + 104xy$
17) $10x^2 - 45y^2$
18) $-6x^3y + 9xy$
19) $-4x^2 + 4xy - 4$
20) $3x^2 - 12xy - 24$
21) $4x^3 - 6x^2y + 4x^2$
22) $x^3 + 5x^2 - 4x^2y$
23) $9x^2 + 9xy - 72y^2$
24) $6x^3 - 9x^2 + 24x$
25) $40x^2 - 160x - 100$
26) $-x^4 + 3x^3 + 7x^2$
27) $x^5 - 2x^4 + 12x^3$
28) $18x^5 - 12x^4 + 12x^3$
29) $24x^4 - 40x^3y + 56x^2y^2$
30) $6x^4 - 10x^3 + 24x^2$
31) $4x^5 + 10x^4 - 8x^3$
32) $30x^3 - 25x^2y + 10xy^2$

Multiplying Binomials

1) $x^2 + 4x + 4$
2) $x^2 - x - 6$
3) $x^2 - 6x + 8$
4) $x^2 + 5x + 6$
5) $x^2 - 9x + 20$
6) $x^2 + 7x + 10$
7) $x^2 - 3x - 18$
8) $x^2 - 12x + 32$
9) $x^2 + 10x + 16$
10) $x^2 + 2x - 8$
11) $x^2 + 8x + 6$
12) $x^2 + 10x + 25$
13) $x^2 - 9$
14) $x^2 - 4$
15) $x^2 + 6x + 9$
16) $x^2 + 10x + 24$
17) $x^2 - 49$
18) $x^2 - 5x - 14$
19) $2x^2 + 8x + 6$
20) $4x^2 + 2x - 12$
21) $2x^2 - 8x - 64$
22) $x^2 - 13x + 42$
23) $x^2 - 64$
24) $12x^2 - 2x - 4$
25) $2x^2 + 9x - 35$
26) $15x^2 + 3x - 12$
27) $24x^2 + 90x + 81$
28) $10x^2 - 18x - 36$
29) $4x^2 + 8x - 32$
30) $36x^2 - 16$
31) $9x^2 - 3x - 12$
32) $x^4 - 4$

Factoring Trinomials

1) $(x+3)(x+5)$
2) $(x-2)(x-3)$
3) $(x+4)(x+2)$
4) $(x-2)(x-4)$
5) $(x-4)(x-4)$
6) $(x-3)(x-4)$
7) $(x+2)(x+9)$
8) $(x+6)(x-4)$
9) $(x-2)(x+6)$
10) $(x-1)(x-9)$
11) $(x-2)(x+7)$
12) $(x-9)(x+3)$
13) $(x+3)(x-14)$
14) $(x+11)(x+11)$
15) $(2x+3)(3x-4)$
16) $(x-15)(x-2)$
17) $(3x-1)(x+4)$
18) $(5x-1)(2x+7)$
19) $(x+12)(x+12)$
20) $(4x-1)(2x+3)$
21) $(x+6)$
22) $(4x-3)$
23) $(3x+2)$

Operations with Polynomials

1) $54x+18$
2) $24x+56$
3) $30x-5$
4) $-24x+9$
5) $18x^3-15x^2$
6) $35x^3-10x^2$
7) $-18x^4+24x^3$
8) $-14x^5+28x^4$
9) $8x^2+16x-24$
10) $16x^2-8x+4$
11) $6x^2+4x-4$
12) $40x^3+24x^2+64x$
13) $27x^2-6x-1$
14) $24x^2+10x-25$
15) $35x^2+27x-18$
16) $9x^2+12x-32$
17) $(5x+4y)$
18) $8x^2+2x-10$
19) $36x^2+108x+81$
20) $34x$
21) $x^3+6x^2+12x+6$
22) $(6x+3y)$

Chapter 9:

Functions Operations

Topics that you'll practice in this chapter:

✓ Evaluating Function
✓ Adding and Subtracting Functions
✓ Multiplying and Dividing Functions
✓ Composition of Functions

Mathematics is like checkers in being suitable for the young, not too difficult, amusing, and without peril to the state. — Plato

Evaluating Function

✎ **Write each of following in function notation.**

1) $h = 2x + 5$

2) $k = 12a - 9$

3) $d = 22t$

4) $y = 2x - 6$

5) $m = 25n - 120$

6) $c = p^2 + 5p + 5$

✎ **Evaluate each function.**

7) $f(x) = x - 2$, find $f(1)$

8) $g(x) = 2x + 3$, find $f(2)$

9) $h(x) = x + 8$, find $f(5)$

10) $f(x) = -x + 5$, find $f(4)$

11) $f(a) = 3a - 3$, find $f(-1)$

12) $h(x) = 12 - 2x$, find $f(6)$

13) $g(n) = 4n - 2$, find $f(-2)$

14) $f(x) = -5x + 3$, find $f(3)$

15) $k(n) = -8 + 4n$, find $f(2)$

16) $f(x) = -7x + 4$, find $f(-3)$

17) $g(n) = 10n - 3$, find $g(6)$

18) $g(n) = 8n + 4$, find $g(1)$

19) $h(x) = 4x - 22$, find $h(2)$

20) $h(n) = n^2 + 2$, find $h(3)$

21) $h(n) = n^2 - 7$, find $h(2)$

22) $h(n) = n^2 + 4$, find $h(-4)$

23) $h(n) = n^2 - 10$, find $h(5)$

24) $h(n) = -2n^2 - 6n$, find $h(2)$

25) $g(n) = 3n^2 + 2n$, find $g(2)$

26) $h(a) = -11a + 5$, find $h(2a)$

27) $k(a) = 7a + 3$, find $k(a - 2)$

28) $h(x) = 3x + 5$, find $h(6x)$

29) $h(x) = x^2 + 1$, find $h(\frac{x}{4})$

30) $h(x) = x^3 + 8$, find $h(3x)$

Adding and Subtracting Functions

✎ **Perform the indicated operation.**

1) $f(x) = 2x + 4$
   $g(x) = x + 3$
   Find $(f - g)(1)$

2) $g(a) = 2a - 1$
   $f(a) = -a - 4$
   Find $(g - f)(-1)$

3) $h(t) = 2t + 1$
   $g(t) = 2t + 2$
   Find $(h - g)(t)$

4) $g(a) = -3a - 3$
   $f(a) = a^2 + 5$
   Find $(g - f)(a)$

5) $g(x) = 2x - 5$
   $h(x) = 4x + 5$
   Find $g(3) - h(3)$

6) $h(3) = 3x + 3$
   $g(x) = -4x + 1$
   Find $(h + g)(10)$

7) $f(x) = 4x - 3$
   $g(x) = x^3 + 2x$
   Find $(f - g)(4)$

8) $h(n) = 4n + 5$
   $g(n) = 3n + 4$
   Find $(h - g)(n)$

9) $g(x) = -x^2 - 1 - 2x$
   $f(x) = 5 + x$
   Find $(g - f)(x)$

10) $g(t) = 2t + 5$
    $f(t) = -t^2 + 5$
    Find $(g + f)(t)$

11) $f(x) = 3x + 2$
    $g(x) = -2x^2 + x$
    Find $(f + g)(x)$

12) $f(x) = -2x^2 - 4x$
    $g(x) = 4x + 3$
    Find $(f + g)(x^2)$

Multiplying and Dividing Functions

✎ **Perform the indicated operation.**

1) $g(x) = -x - 2$
   $f(x) = 2x + 1$
   Find $(g.f)(2)$

2) $f(x) = 3x$
   $h(x) = -2x + 5$
   Find $(f.h)(-1)$

3) $g(a) = 2a - 1$
   $h(a) = 3a - 3$
   Find $(g.h)(-4)$

4) $f(x) = x + 4$
   $h(x) = 5x - 2$
   Find $\left(\frac{f}{h}\right)(2)$

5) $f(x) = 2a^2$
   $g(x) = -5 + 3a$
   Find $\left(\frac{f}{g}\right)(2)$

6) $g(a) = 3a + 2$
   $f(a) = 2a - 4$
   Find $\left(\frac{g}{f}\right)(3)$

7) $g(t) = t^2 + 3$
   $h(t) = 4t - 3$
   Find $(g.h)(-1)$

8) $g(n) = n^2 + 4 + 2n$
   $h(n) = -3n + 2$
   Find $(g.h)(1)$

9) $g(a) = 2a^3 - 5a + 2$
   $f(a) = a^3 - 4$
   Find $\left(\frac{g}{f}\right)(2)$

10) $g(x) = -2x^2 + 14 - 2x$
    $f(x) = x^2 + 5$
    Find $(g.f)(4)$

11) $f(x) = 2x^3 - 5x^2$
    $g(x) = 2x - 1$
    Find $(f.g)(x)$

12) $f(x) = 3x - 1$
    $g(x) = x^2 - x$
    Find $\left(\frac{f}{g}\right)(x)$

Composition of Functions

✎ **Using** f(x) = x + 2 **and** g(x) = 4x, **find:**

1) $f(g(1)) =$

2) $f(g(-2)) =$

3) $g(f(-1)) =$

4) $g(f(3)) =$

5) $f(g(2)) =$

6) $g(f(5)) =$

✎ **Using** f(x) = 5x + 4 **and** g(x) = x − 3, **find:**

7) $g(f(-3)) =$

8) $g(f(4)) =$

9) $f(g(6)) =$

10) $f(f(8)) =$

11) $g(f(-7)) =$

12) $g(f(x)) =$

✎ **Using** f(x) = 6x + 2 **and** g(x) = x − 5, **find:**

13) $g(f(-2)) =$

14) $f(f(4)) =$

15) $f(g(7)) =$

16) $f(f(2)) =$

17) $g(f(3)) =$

18) $g(g(x)) =$

✎ **Using** f(x) = 7x + 4 **and** g(x) = 2x − 4, **find:**

19) $f(g(-3)) =$

20) $g(f(-2)) =$

21) $f(g(3)) =$

22) $f(f(3)) =$

23) $g(f(4)) =$

24) $g(g(5)) =$

Answers of Worksheets – Chapter 9

Evaluating Function

1) $h(x) = 2x + 5$
2) $k(a) = 12a - 9$
3) $d(t) = 22t$
4) $f(x) = 2x - 6$
5) $m(n) = 25n - 120$
6) $c(p) = p^2 + 5p + 5$
7) -1
8) 7
9) 13
10) 1
11) -6
12) 0
13) -10
14) -12
15) 0
16) 25
17) 57
18) 12
19) -14
20) 11
21) -3
22) 20
23) 15
24) -20
25) 16
26) $-22a + 5$
27) $7a - 11$
28) $18x + 5$
29) $\frac{1}{16}x^2 + 1$
30) $27x^3 + 8$

Adding and Subtracting Functions

1) 2
2) 0
3) -1
4) $-a^2 - 3a - 8$
5) -16
6) -6
7) -59
8) $n + 1$
9) $-x^2 - 3x - 6$
10) $-t^2 + 2t + 10$
11) $-2x^2 + 4x + 2$
12) $-2x^6 + 3$

Multiplying and Dividing Functions

1) -20
2) -21
3) 135
4) $\frac{6}{8} = \frac{3}{4}$
5) 8
6) $\frac{11}{2}$
7) -28
8) -7
9) 2
10) -546
11) $4x^4 - 12x^3 + 5x^2$
12) $\frac{3x-1}{x^2-x}$

Composition of Functions

1) 6
2) −6
3) 4
4) 20
5) 10
6) 28
7) −14
8) 24
9) 19
10) 41
11) −31
12) $5x + 1$
13) −15
14) 21
15) 14
16) 86
17) 15
18) $x - 10$
19) −66
20) −24
21) 18
22) 179
23) 60
24) 8

Chapter 10:

Quadratic

Topics that you'll practice in this chapter:

✓ Graphing Quadratic Functions

✓ Solving Quadratic Equations

✓ Use the Quadratic Formula and the Discriminant

✓ Solve Quadratic Inequalities

It's fine to work on any problem, so long as it generates interesting Mathematics along the way – even if you don't solve it at the end of the day." – Andrew Wiles

Solving Quadratic Equations

✎ **Solve each equation by factoring or using the quadratic formula.**

1) $(x + 2)(x - 7) = 0$

2) $(x + 3)(x + 5) = 0$

3) $(x - 9)(x + 4) = 0$

4) $(x - 7)(x - 5) = 0$

5) $(x + 4)(x + 8) = 0$

6) $(5x + 7)(x + 4) = 0$

7) $(2x + 5)(4x + 3) = 0$

8) $(3x + 4)(x + 2) = 0$

9) $(6x + 3)(2x + 4) = 0$

10) $(9x + 3)(x + 6) = 0$

11) $x^2 = 2x$

12) $x^2 - 6 = x$

13) $2x^2 + 4 = 6x$

14) $-x^2 - 6 = 5x$

15) $x^2 + 8x = 9$

16) $x^2 + 10x = 24$

17) $x^2 + 7x = -10$

18) $x^2 + 12x = -32$

19) $x^2 + 11x = -28$

20) $x^2 + x - 20 = 2x$

21) $x^2 + 8x = -15$

22) $7x^2 - 14x = -7$

23) $10x^2 = 27x - 18$

24) $7x^2 - 6x + 3 = 3$

25) $2x^2 - 14 = -3x$

26) $10x^2 - 26x = -12$

27) $15x^2 + 80 = -80x$

28) $x^2 + 15x = -56$

29) $6x^2 - 18x - 18 = 6$

30) $2x^2 + 6x - 24 = 12$

31) $2x^2 - 22x + 38 = -10$

32) $-4x^2 - 8x - 3 = -3 - 5x^2$

Quadratic Formula and the Discriminant

✍ *Find the value of the discriminant of each quadratic equation.*

1) $x(x-1) = 0$

2) $x^2 + 2x - 1 = 0$

3) $x^2 + 3x + 5 = 0$

4) $x^2 - x + 4 = 0$

5) $x^2 + x - 2 = 0$

6) $x^2 + 4x - 6 = 0$

7) $x^2 + 5x + 2 = 0$

8) $2x^2 - 2x - 7 = 0$

9) $2x^2 + 3x + 9 = 0$

10) $2x^2 + 5x - 4 = 0$

11) $5x^2 + x - 2 = 0$

12) $-3x^2 - 6x + 2 = 0$

13) $-4x^2 - 4x + 5 = 0$

14) $-2x^2 - x - 1 = 0$

15) $6x^2 - 2x - 3 = 0$

16) $-5x^2 - 3x + 9 = 0$

17) $4x^2 + 5x - 4 = 0$

18) $8x^2 - 9x = 0$

19) $3x^2 - 5x + 1 = 0$

20) $5x^2 + 6x + 4 = 0$

✍ *Find the discriminant of each quadratic equation then state the number of real and imaginary solutions.*

21) $-x^2 - 9 = 6x$

22) $4x^2 = 8x - 4$

23) $-4x^2 - 4x = 6$

24) $8x^2 - 6x + 3 = 5x^2$

25) $-9x^2 = -8x + 8$

26) $9x^2 + 6x + 6 = 5$

27) $9x^2 - 3x - 8 = -10$

28) $-2x^2 - 8x - 14 = -6$

Quadratic Inequalities

✎ **Solve each quadratic inequality.**

1) $x^2 - 1 < 0$

2) $-x^2 - 5x + 6 > 0$

3) $x^2 - 5x - 6 < 0$

4) $x^2 + 4x - 5 > 0$

5) $x^2 - 2x - 3 \geq 0$

6) $x^2 > 5x + 6$

7) $-x^2 - 12x - 11 \leq 0$

8) $x^2 - 2x - 8 \geq 0$

9) $x^2 - 5x - 6 \geq 0$

10) $x^2 + 7x + 10 < 0$

11) $x^2 + 9x + 20 > 0$

12) $x^2 - 8x + 16 > 0$

13) $x^2 - 8x + 12 \leq 0$

14) $x^2 - 11x + 30 \leq 0$

15) $x^2 - 12x + 27 \geq 0$

16) $x^2 - 16x + 64 \geq 0$

17) $x^2 - 36 \leq 0$

18) $x^2 - 13x + 36 \geq 0$

19) $x^2 + 15x + 36 \leq 0$

20) $4x^2 - 6x - 9 > x^2$

21) $5x^2 - 15x + 10 < 0$

22) $3x^2 - 5x \geq 4x^2 + 6$

23) $4x^2 - 12 > 3x^2 + x$

24) $x^2 - 2x \geq x^2 - 6x + 12$

25) $2x^2 + 2x - 8 > x^2$

26) $4x^2 + 20x - 11 < 0$

27) $-9x^2 + 29x - 6 \geq 0$

28) $-8x^2 + 6x - 1 \leq 0$

29) $12x^2 + 10x - 12 > 0$

30) $18x^2 + 23x + 5 \leq 0$

31) $17x^2 + 15x - 2 \geq 0$

32) $3x^2 + 7x \leq 5x^2 + 3x - 6$

Graphing Quadratic Functions

✎ *Sketch the graph of each function. Identify the vertex and axis of symmetry.*

1) $y = 3(x + 1)^2 + 2$

2) $y = -(x - 2)^2 - 4$

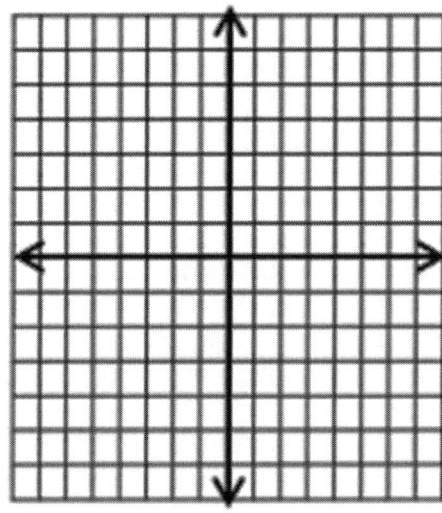
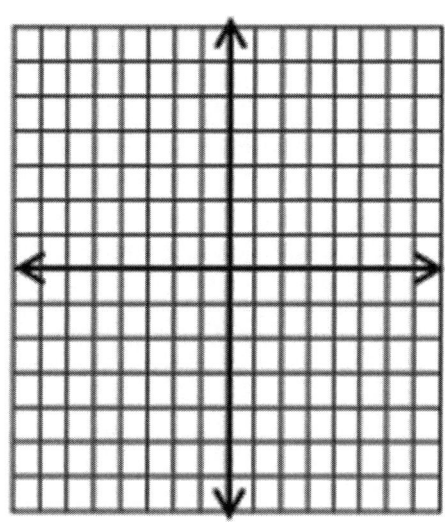

3) $y = 2(x - 3)^2 + 8$

4) $y = x^2 - 8x + 19$

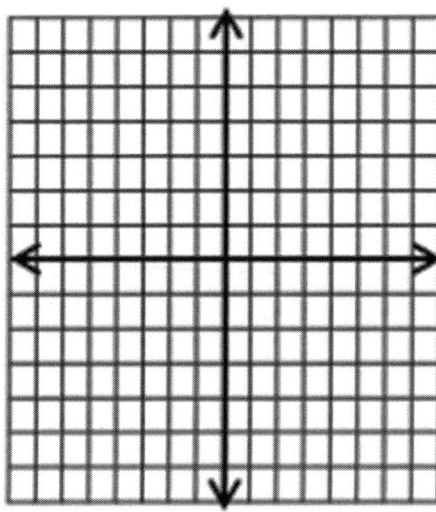
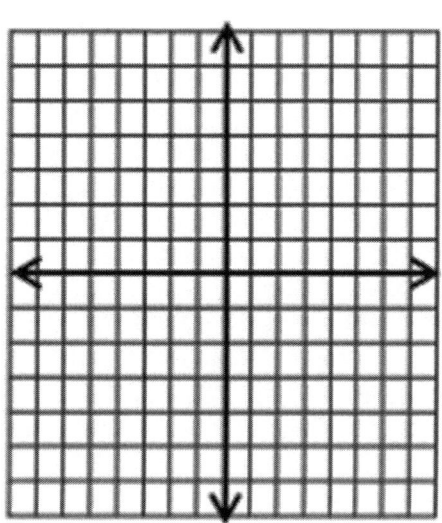

Answers of Worksheets – Chapter 10

Solving quadratic equations

1) $\{-2, 7\}$
2) $\{-3, -5\}$
3) $\{9, -4\}$
4) $\{7, 5\}$
5) $\{-4, -8\}$
6) $\{-\frac{7}{5}, -4\}$
7) $\{-\frac{5}{2}, -\frac{3}{4}\}$
8) $\{-\frac{4}{3}, -2\}$
9) $\{-\frac{1}{2}, -2\}$
10) $\{-\frac{1}{3}, -6\}$

11) $\{2, 0\}$
12) $\{3, -2\}$
13) $\{2, 1\}$
14) $\{-3, -2\}$
15) $\{1, -9\}$
16) $\{2, -12\}$
17) $\{-2, -5\}$
18) $\{-4, -8\}$
19) $\{-4, -7\}$
20) $\{5, -4\}$
21) $\{-5, -3\}$
22) $\{1\}$

23) $\{\frac{6}{5}, \frac{3}{2}\}$
24) $\{\frac{6}{7}, 0\}$
25) $\{-\frac{7}{2}, 2\}$
26) $\{\frac{3}{5}, 2\}$
27) $\{-\frac{4}{3}, -4\}$
28) $\{-8, -7\}$
29) $\{4, -1\}$
30) $\{3, -6\}$
31) $\{3, 8\}$
32) $\{8, 0\}$

Quadratic formula and the discriminant

1) 1
2) 8
3) -11
4) -15
5) 9
6) 40
7) 17
8) 60
9) -45
10) 57

11) 41
12) 60
13) 96
14) -7
15) 76
16) 189
17) 89
18) 81
19) 13
20) -44

21) 0, one real solution
22) 0, one real solution
23) -80, no solution
24) 0, one real solution
25) -224, no solution
26) 0, one real solution
27) -63, solution
28) 0, one real solution

Solve quadratic inequalities

1) $-1 < x < 1$
2) $-6 < x < 1$
3) $-1 < x < 6$
4) $x < -5 \text{ or } x > 1$
5) $x \leq -1 \text{ or } x \geq 3$
6) $x < -1 \text{ or } x > 6$
7) $x \leq -11 \text{ or } x \geq -1$
8) $x \leq -2 \text{ or } x \geq 4$
9) $x \leq -1 \text{ or } x \geq 6$
10) $-5 < x < -2$
11) $x < -5 \text{ or } x > -4$
12) $x < 4 \text{ or } x > 4$

13) $2 \leq x \leq 6$
14) $5 \leq x \leq 6$
15) $x \leq 3 \text{ or } x \geq 9$
16) all real numbers
17) $-6 \leq x \leq 6$
18) $x \leq 4 \text{ or } x \geq 9$
19) $-12 \leq x \leq -3$
20) $x < -1 \text{ or } x > 3$
21) $1 < x < 2$
22) $-3 \leq x \leq -2$
23) $x < -3 \text{ or } x > 4$
24) $x \geq 3$

25) $x < -4 \text{ or } x > 2$
26) $-\frac{11}{2} < x < \frac{1}{2}$
27) $\frac{2}{9} \leq x \leq 3$
28) $x \leq \frac{1}{4} \text{ or } x \geq \frac{1}{2}$
29) $x < -1.5 \text{ or } x > \frac{2}{3}$
30) $-1 \leq x \leq -\frac{5}{18}$
31) $x \leq -1 \text{ or } x \geq \frac{2}{17}$
32) $x \leq -1 \text{ or } x \geq 3$

Graphing quadratic functions

1) $(-1, 2), x = -1$

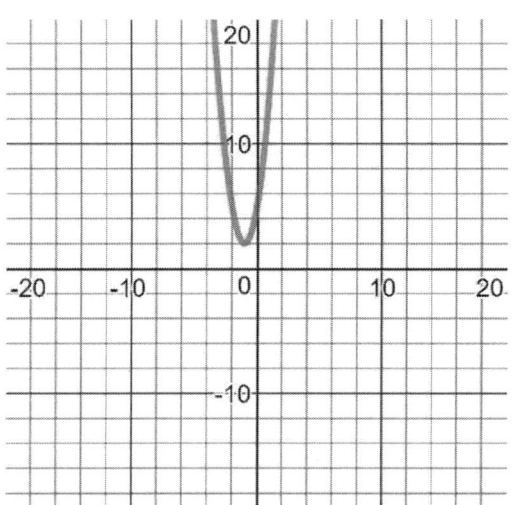

2) $(2, -4), x = 2$

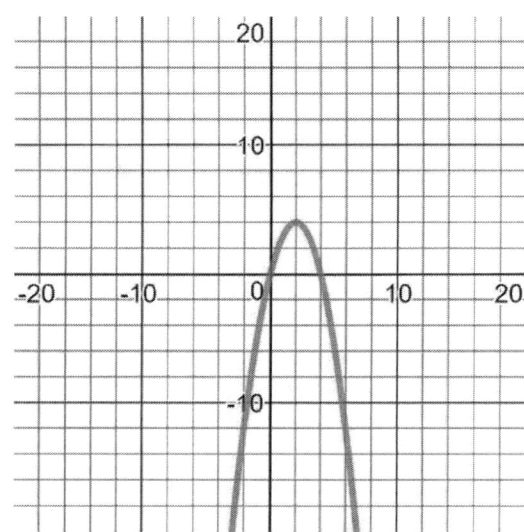

3) $(3, 8), x = 3$

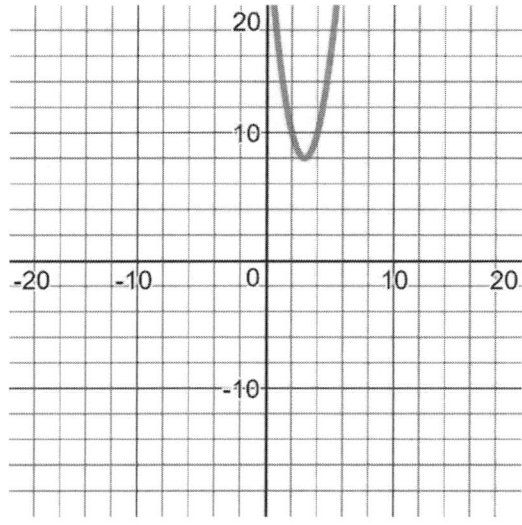

4) $(4, 3), x = 4$

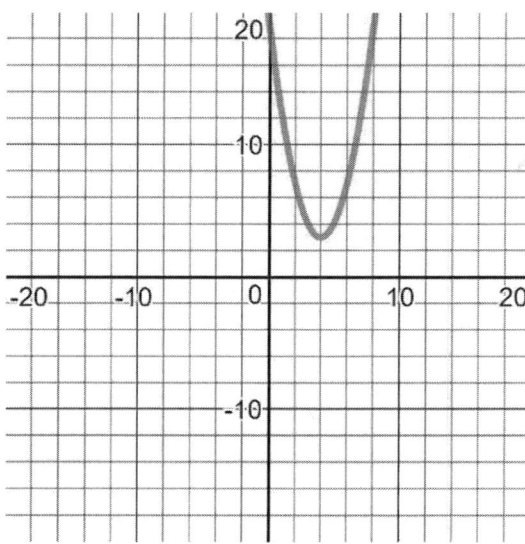

Chapter 11:

Radical Expressions

Topics that you'll practice in this chapter:

- ✓ Simplifying Radical Expressions
- ✓ Simplifying Radical Expressions Involving Fractions
- ✓ Multiplying Radical Expressions
- ✓ Adding and Subtracting Radical Expressions
- ✓ Domain and Range of Radical Functions
- ✓ Solving Radical Equations

Mathematics is an independent world created out of pure intelligence.

— *William Woods Worth*

Simplifying Radical Expressions

✎ **Simplify.**

1) $\sqrt{35x^2} =$

2) $\sqrt{90x^2} =$

3) $\sqrt[3]{8a} =$

4) $\sqrt{100x^3} =$

5) $\sqrt{125a} =$

6) $\sqrt[3]{88w^3} =$

7) $\sqrt{80x} =$

8) $\sqrt{216v} =$

9) $\sqrt[3]{125x} =$

10) $\sqrt{64x^5} =$

11) $\sqrt{4x^2} =$

12) $\sqrt[3]{54a^2} =$

13) $\sqrt{405} =$

14) $\sqrt{512p^3} =$

15) $\sqrt{216m^4} =$

16) $\sqrt{264x^3y^3} =$

17) $\sqrt{49x^3y^3} =$

18) $\sqrt{16a^4b^3} =$

19) $\sqrt{20x^3y^3} =$

20) $\sqrt[3]{216yx^3} =$

21) $3\sqrt{75x^2} =$

22) $5\sqrt{80x^2} =$

23) $\sqrt[3]{256x^2y^3} =$

24) $\sqrt[3]{343x^4y^2} =$

25) $4\sqrt{125a} =$

26) $\sqrt[3]{625xy} =$

27) $2\sqrt{8x^2y^3r} =$

28) $4\sqrt{36x^2y^3z^4} =$

29) $2\sqrt[3]{512x^3y^4} =$

30) $5\sqrt{64a^2b^3c^5} =$

31) $2\sqrt[3]{125x^6y^{12}} =$

Multiplying Radical Expressions

✎ Simplify.

1) $\sqrt{5} \times \sqrt{5} =$

2) $\sqrt{5} \times \sqrt{10} =$

3) $\sqrt{2} \times \sqrt{18} =$

4) $\sqrt{14} \times \sqrt{21} =$

5) $\sqrt{5} \times -4\sqrt{20} =$

6) $3\sqrt{12} \times \sqrt{6} =$

7) $5\sqrt{42} \times \sqrt{3} =$

8) $\sqrt{3} \times -\sqrt{25} =$

9) $\sqrt{99} \times \sqrt{48} =$

10) $5\sqrt{45} \times 3\sqrt{176} =$

11) $\sqrt{12}(3 + \sqrt{3}) =$

12) $\sqrt{23x^2} \times \sqrt{23x} =$

13) $-5\sqrt{12} \times -\sqrt{3} =$

14) $2\sqrt{20x^2} \times \sqrt{5x^2} =$

15) $\sqrt{12x^2} \times \sqrt{2x^3} =$

16) $-12\sqrt{7x} \times \sqrt{5x^3} =$

17) $-5\sqrt{9x^3} \times 6\sqrt{3x^2} =$

18) $-2\sqrt{12}(3 + \sqrt{12}) =$

19) $\sqrt{18x}\,(4 - \sqrt{6x}) =$

20) $\sqrt{3x}(6\sqrt{x^3} + \sqrt{27}) =$

21) $\sqrt{15r}\,(5 + \sqrt{5}) =$

22) $-5\sqrt{3x} \times 4\sqrt{6x^3} =$

23) $-2\sqrt{18x} \times 4\sqrt{2x}$

24) $-3\sqrt{5v^2}\,(-3\sqrt{15v}) =$

25) $(\sqrt{5} - \sqrt{3})(\sqrt{5} + \sqrt{3}) =$

26) $(-4\sqrt{6} + 2)(\sqrt{6} - 5) =$

27) $(2 - 2\sqrt{3})(-2 + \sqrt{3}) =$

28) $(11 - 4\sqrt{5})(6 - \sqrt{5}) =$

29) $(-2 - \sqrt{3x})(3 + \sqrt{3x}) =$

30) $(-2 + 3\sqrt{2r})(-2 + \sqrt{2r}) =$

31) $(-4\sqrt{2n} + 2)(-2\sqrt{2} - 4) =$

32) $(-1 + 2\sqrt{3})(2 - 3\sqrt{3x}) =$

Simplifying Radical Expressions Involving Fractions

✎ *Simplify.*

1) $\dfrac{\sqrt{5}}{\sqrt{3}} =$

2) $\dfrac{\sqrt{8}}{\sqrt{100}} =$

3) $\dfrac{\sqrt{2}}{2\sqrt{3}} =$

4) $\dfrac{4}{\sqrt{5}} =$

5) $\dfrac{2\sqrt{5r}}{\sqrt{m^3}} =$

6) $\dfrac{8\sqrt{3}}{\sqrt{k}} =$

7) $\dfrac{6\sqrt{14x^2}}{2\sqrt{18x}} =$

8) $\dfrac{\sqrt{7x^2y^2}}{\sqrt{5x^3y^2}} =$

9) $\dfrac{1}{1+\sqrt{2}} =$

10) $\dfrac{1-5\sqrt{a}}{\sqrt{11a}} =$

11) $\dfrac{\sqrt{a}}{\sqrt{a}+\sqrt{b}} =$

12) $\dfrac{1+\sqrt{2}}{3+\sqrt{5}} =$

13) $\dfrac{2+\sqrt{5}}{6-\sqrt{3}} =$

14) $\dfrac{5}{-3-3\sqrt{3}} =$

15) $\dfrac{2}{3+\sqrt{5}} =$

16) $\dfrac{\sqrt{7}-\sqrt{3}}{\sqrt{3}-\sqrt{7}} =$

17) $\dfrac{\sqrt{7}+\sqrt{5}}{\sqrt{5}+\sqrt{2}} =$

18) $\dfrac{3\sqrt{2}-\sqrt{7}}{4\sqrt{2}+\sqrt{5}} =$

19) $\dfrac{\sqrt{5}+2\sqrt{2}}{4-\sqrt{5}} =$

20) $\dfrac{5\sqrt{3}-3\sqrt{2}}{3\sqrt{2}-2\sqrt{3}} =$

21) $\dfrac{\sqrt{8a^5b^3}}{\sqrt{2ab^2}} =$

22) $\dfrac{6\sqrt{45x^3}}{3\sqrt{5x}} =$

Adding and Subtracting Radical Expressions

✎ Simplify.

1) $\sqrt{3} + \sqrt{27} =$

2) $3\sqrt{8} + 3\sqrt{2} =$

3) $4\sqrt{3} - 2\sqrt{12} =$

4) $3\sqrt{18} - 2\sqrt{2} =$

5) $2\sqrt{45} - 2\sqrt{5} =$

6) $-\sqrt{12} - 5\sqrt{3} =$

7) $-4\sqrt{2} - 5\sqrt{32} =$

8) $5\sqrt{10} + 2\sqrt{40} =$

9) $4\sqrt{12} - 3\sqrt{27} =$

10) $-3\sqrt{2} + 4\sqrt{18} =$

11) $-10\sqrt{7} + 6\sqrt{28} =$

12) $5\sqrt{3} - \sqrt{27} =$

13) $-\sqrt{12} + 3\sqrt{3} =$

14) $-3\sqrt{6} - \sqrt{54} =$

15) $3\sqrt{8} + 3\sqrt{2} =$

16) $2\sqrt{12} - 3\sqrt{27} =$

17) $\sqrt{50} - \sqrt{32} =$

18) $4\sqrt{8} - 6\sqrt{2} =$

19) $-4\sqrt{12} + 12\sqrt{108} =$

20) $2\sqrt{45} - 2\sqrt{5} =$

21) $7\sqrt{18} - 3\sqrt{2} =$

22) $-12\sqrt{35} + 7\sqrt{140} =$

23) $-6\sqrt{19} - 3\sqrt{76} =$

24) $-\sqrt{54x} - 3\sqrt{6x} =$

25) $\sqrt{5y^2} + y\sqrt{45} =$

26) $\sqrt{8mn^2} + 2n\sqrt{18m} =$

27) $-8\sqrt{27a} - 5\sqrt{3a} =$

28) $-4\sqrt{7ab} - \sqrt{28ab} =$

29) $\sqrt{27a^2b} + a\sqrt{12b} =$

30) $3\sqrt{6a^3} - 2\sqrt{24a^3} + 2a\sqrt{54a} =$

Domain and Range of Radical Functions

✎ **Identify the domain and range of each function.**

1) $y = \sqrt{x+2} - 3$

2) $y = \sqrt[3]{x-1} - 1$

3) $y = \sqrt{x-2} + 5$

4) $y = \sqrt[3]{(x+1)} - 4$

5) $y = 3\sqrt{3x+6} + 5$

6) $y = \sqrt[3]{(2x-1)} - 4$

7) $y = 6\sqrt{3x^2+6} + 5$

8) $y = \sqrt[3]{(2x^2-2)} - 4$

9) $y = 4\sqrt{4x^3+32} - 1$

10) $y = \sqrt[3]{(4x+8)} - 2x$

11) $y = 7\sqrt{-2(2x+4)} + 1$

12) $y = \sqrt[5]{(4x^2-5)} - 2$

13) $y = 2x\sqrt{5x^4+6} - 2x$

14) $y = 6\sqrt[3]{(8x^6+2x+8)} - 2$

✎ **Sketch the graph of each function.**

5) $y = \sqrt{x} + 8$

6) $y = 2\sqrt{x} - 4$

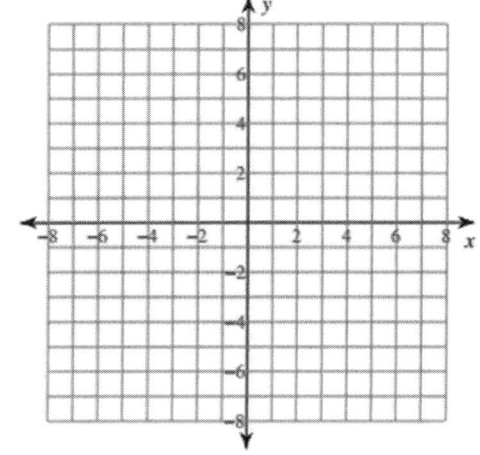
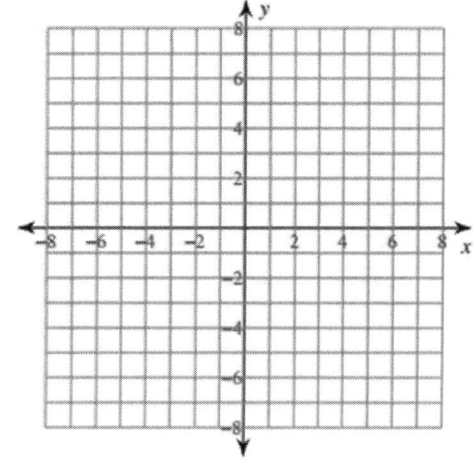

Solving Radical Equations

✎ **Solve each equation. Remember to check for extraneous solutions.**

1) $\sqrt{a} = 5$

2) $\sqrt{v} = 3$

3) $\sqrt{r} = 4$

4) $2 = 4\sqrt{x}$

5) $\sqrt{x+1} = 9$

6) $1 = \sqrt{x-5}$

7) $6 = \sqrt{r-2}$

8) $\sqrt{x-6} = 8$

9) $5 = \sqrt{x-3}$

10) $\sqrt{m+8} = 8$

11) $10\sqrt{9a} = 60$

12) $5\sqrt{3x} = 15$

13) $1 = \sqrt{3x-5}$

14) $\sqrt{12-x} = x$

15) $\sqrt{r+3} - 1 = 7$

16) $-12 = -6\sqrt{r+4}$

17) $20 = 2\sqrt{36v}$

18) $x = \sqrt{42-x}$

19) $\sqrt{110-a} = a$

20) $\sqrt{2n-12} = 2$

21) $\sqrt{3r-5} = r-3$

22) $\sqrt{-16+10x} = x$

23) $\sqrt{3x+12} = \sqrt{x+8}$

24) $\sqrt{v} = \sqrt{2v-6}$

25) $\sqrt{11-x} = \sqrt{x-7}$

26) $\sqrt{m+8} = \sqrt{3m+8}$

27) $\sqrt{2r+40} = \sqrt{-16-2r}$

28) $\sqrt{k+3} = \sqrt{1-k}$

29) $-10\sqrt{x-10} = -60$

30) $\sqrt{72-x} = \sqrt{\dfrac{x}{5}}$

Answers of Worksheets – Chapter 11

Simplifying radical expressions

1) $x\sqrt{35}$
2) $3x\sqrt{10}$
3) $2\sqrt[3]{a}$
4) $10x\sqrt{x}$
5) $5\sqrt{5a}$
6) $2w\sqrt[3]{11}$
7) $4\sqrt{5x}$
8) $6\sqrt{6v}$
9) $5\sqrt[3]{x}$
10) $8x^2\sqrt{x}$
11) $2x$
12) $3\sqrt[3]{2a^2}$
13) $9\sqrt{5}$
14) $16p\sqrt{2p}$
15) $6m^2\sqrt{6}$
16) $2x.y\sqrt{66xy}$
17) $7xy\sqrt{xy}$
18) $4a^2b\sqrt{b}$
19) $2xy\sqrt{5xy}$
20) $6x\sqrt[3]{y}$
21) $15x\sqrt{3}$
22) $20x\sqrt{5}$
23) $16y\sqrt[3]{x^2}$
24) $7x\sqrt[3]{xy^2}$
25) $20\sqrt{5a}$
26) $5\sqrt[3]{5xy}$
27) $4xy\sqrt{2yr}$
28) $24\ x\ yz^2\sqrt{y}$
29) $16xy\sqrt[3]{y}$
30) $40abc^2\sqrt{bc}$
31) $10x^2y^4$

Multiplying radical expressions

1) 5
2) $5\sqrt{2}$
3) 6
4) $7\sqrt{6}$
5) -40
6) $18\sqrt{2}$
7) $15\sqrt{14}$
8) $-5\sqrt{3}$
9) $12\sqrt{33}$
10) $180\sqrt{55}$
11) $6\sqrt{3}+6$
12) $23x\sqrt{x}$
13) 30
14) $20x^2$
15) $2x\sqrt{6x}$
16) $-12x^2\sqrt{35}$
17) $-90x^2\sqrt{3x}$
18) $-12\sqrt{3}-24$
19) $6\sqrt{2x}-6x\sqrt{3}$
20) $54x^2$
21) $5\sqrt{15r}+3\sqrt{5r}$
22) $-60x^2\sqrt{2}$
23) $-48x$
24) $45v\sqrt{3v}$

25) 2

26) $22\sqrt{3} - 34$

27) $6\sqrt{3} - 10$

28) $86 - 35\sqrt{5}$

29) $-3x - 5\sqrt{3x} - 6$

30) $12r - 8\sqrt{2r} + 4$

31) $16\sqrt{n} + 16\sqrt{2n} - 4\sqrt{2} - 8$

32) $-2 + 3\sqrt{3x} + 4\sqrt{3} - 18\sqrt{x}$

Simplifying radical expressions involving fractions

1) $\dfrac{\sqrt{15}}{3}$

2) $\dfrac{\sqrt{2}}{5}$

3) $\dfrac{\sqrt{6}}{6}$

4) $\dfrac{4\sqrt{5}}{5}$

5) $\dfrac{2\sqrt{5m}}{m^2}$

6) $\dfrac{8\sqrt{3k}}{k}$

7) $\sqrt{7x}$

8) $\dfrac{\sqrt{35}}{5x}$

9) $-1 + \sqrt{2}$

10) $\dfrac{\sqrt{11a} - 5a\sqrt{11}}{11a}$

11) $\dfrac{a - \sqrt{ab}}{a - b}$

12) $\dfrac{3 - \sqrt{5} + 3\sqrt{2} - \sqrt{10}}{4}$

13) $\dfrac{12 + 2\sqrt{3} + 6\sqrt{5} + \sqrt{15}}{33}$

14) $\dfrac{5 - 5\sqrt{5}}{6}$

15) $-3 + \sqrt{5}$

16) -1

17) $\dfrac{\sqrt{35} - \sqrt{14} + 5 - \sqrt{10}}{3}$

18) $\dfrac{24 - 3\sqrt{10} - 4\sqrt{14} + \sqrt{35}}{27}$

19) $\dfrac{4\sqrt{5} + 5 + 8\sqrt{2} + 2\sqrt{10}}{11}$

20) $\dfrac{3\sqrt{6} + 4}{2}$

21) $2a^2\sqrt{b}$

22) $6x$

Adding and subtracting radical expressions

1) $4\sqrt{3}$

2) $9\sqrt{2}$

3) 0

4) $7\sqrt{2}$

5) $4\sqrt{5}$

6) $-7\sqrt{3}$

7) $-24\sqrt{2}$

8) $9\sqrt{10}$

9) $-\sqrt{3}$

10) $9\sqrt{2}$

11) $2\sqrt{7}$

12) $2\sqrt{3}$

13) $\sqrt{3}$
14) 0
15) $9\sqrt{2}$
16) $-5\sqrt{3}$
17) $\sqrt{2}$
18) $2\sqrt{2}$

19) $64\sqrt{3}$
20) $4\sqrt{5}$
21) $18\sqrt{2}$
22) $2\sqrt{35}$
23) $-12\sqrt{19}$
24) $-6\sqrt{6x}$

25) $4y\sqrt{5}$
26) $8n\sqrt{2m}$
27) $-29\sqrt{3a}$
28) $-8\sqrt{7ab}$
29) $5a\sqrt{3b}$
30) $5a\sqrt{6a}$

Domain and range of radical functions

1) domain: $x \geq -2$
   range: $y \geq -3$

2) domain: {all real numbers}
   range: {all real numbers}

3) domain: $x \geq 2$
   range: $y \geq 5$

4) domain: {all real numbers}
   range: {all real numbers}

5) domain: $x \geq -2$
   range: $y \geq 5$

6) domain: {all real numbers}
   range: {all real numbers}

7) domain: {all real numbers}
   range: {all real numbers}

8) domain: {all real numbers}
   range: {all real numbers}

9) domain: $x \geq -2$
   range: $y \geq -1$

10) domain: {all real numbers}
    range: {all real numbers}

11) domain: $x \leq -2$
    range: $y \geq 1$

12) domain: {all real numbers}
    range: {all real numbers}

13) domain: {all real numbers}
    range: {all real numbers}

14) domain: {all real numbers}
    range: {all real numbers}

5)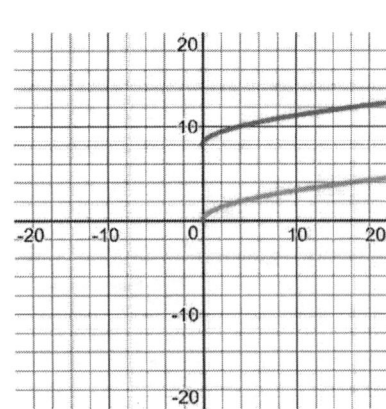

6)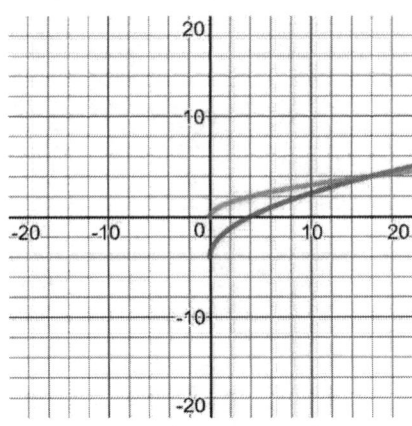

Solving radical equations

1) {25}
2) {9}
3) {16}
4) {$\frac{1}{4}$}
5) {80}
6) {6}
7) {38}
8) {70}
9) {28}
10) {56}

11) {4}
12) {3}
13) {2}
14) {3}
15) {61}
16) {0}
17) {$\frac{25}{9}$}
18) {6}
19) {10}
20) {8}

21) {4}
22) {2, 8}
23) {−2}
24) {6}
25) {9}
26) {0}
27) {−14}
28) {−1}
29) {46}
30) {60}

Chapter 12:

Geometry and Solid Figures

Topics that you'll practice in this chapter:

- ✓ Angles
- ✓ Pythagorean Relationship
- ✓ Triangles
- ✓ Polygons
- ✓ Trapezoids
- ✓ Circles
- ✓ Cubes
- ✓ Rectangular Prism
- ✓ Cylinder
- ✓ Pyramids and Cone

Mathematics is, as it were, a sensuous logic, and relates to philosophy as do the arts, music, and plastic art to poetry. — K. Shegel

Angles

✎ **What is the value of x in the following figures?**

1)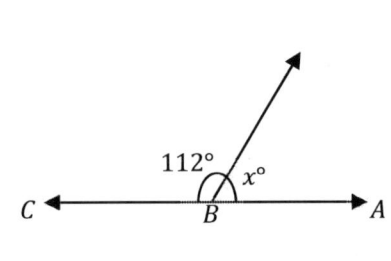

2)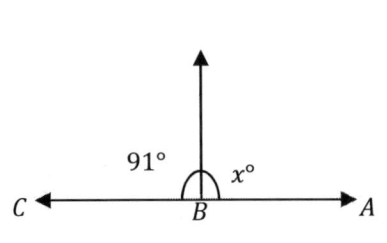

3)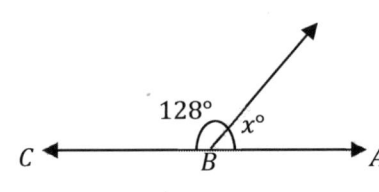

4)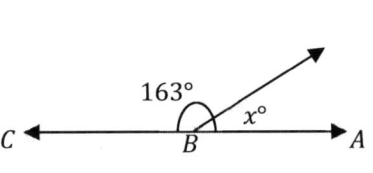

5)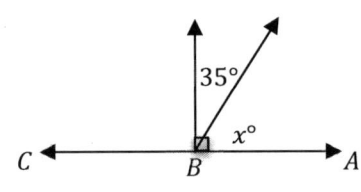

6)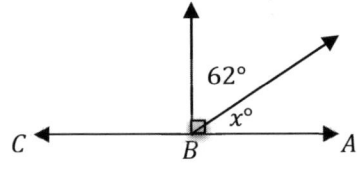

✎ **Solve.**

7) Two complementary angles have equal measures. What is the measure of each angle? _____

8) The measure of an angle is two third the measure of its supplement. What is the measure of the angle? _____

9) Two angles are complementary and the measure of one angle is 24 less than the other. What is the measure of the bigger angle? _____

10) Two angles are complementary. The measure of one angle is half the measure of the other. What is the measure of the smaller angle? _____

11) Two supplementary angles are given. The measure of one angle is 50° less than the measure of the other. What does the bigger angle measure? _____

Pythagorean Relationship

✍ Do the following lengths form a right triangle?

1)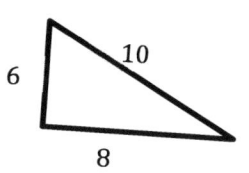

2)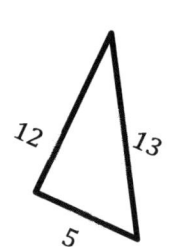

3)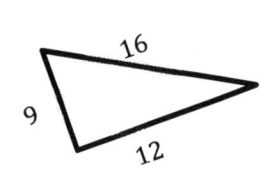

4)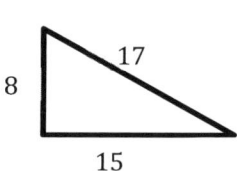

5)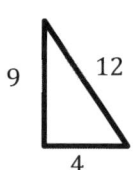

6)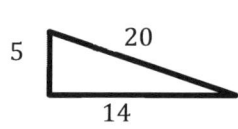

7)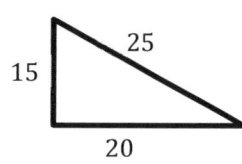

8)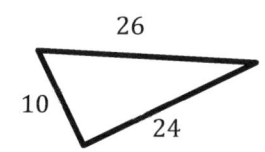

✍ Find the missing side?

9)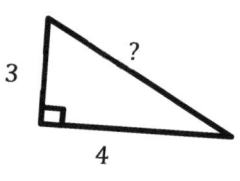

10)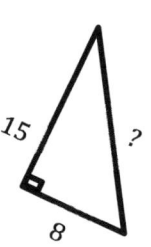

11)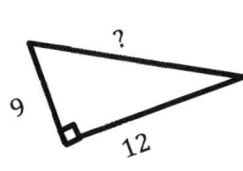

12)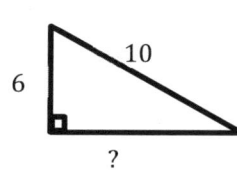

13)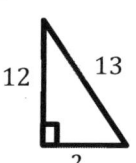

14)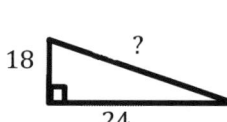

15)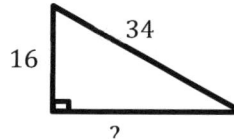

16)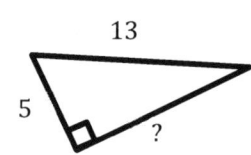

Triangles

✎ **Find the measure of the unknown angle in each triangle.**

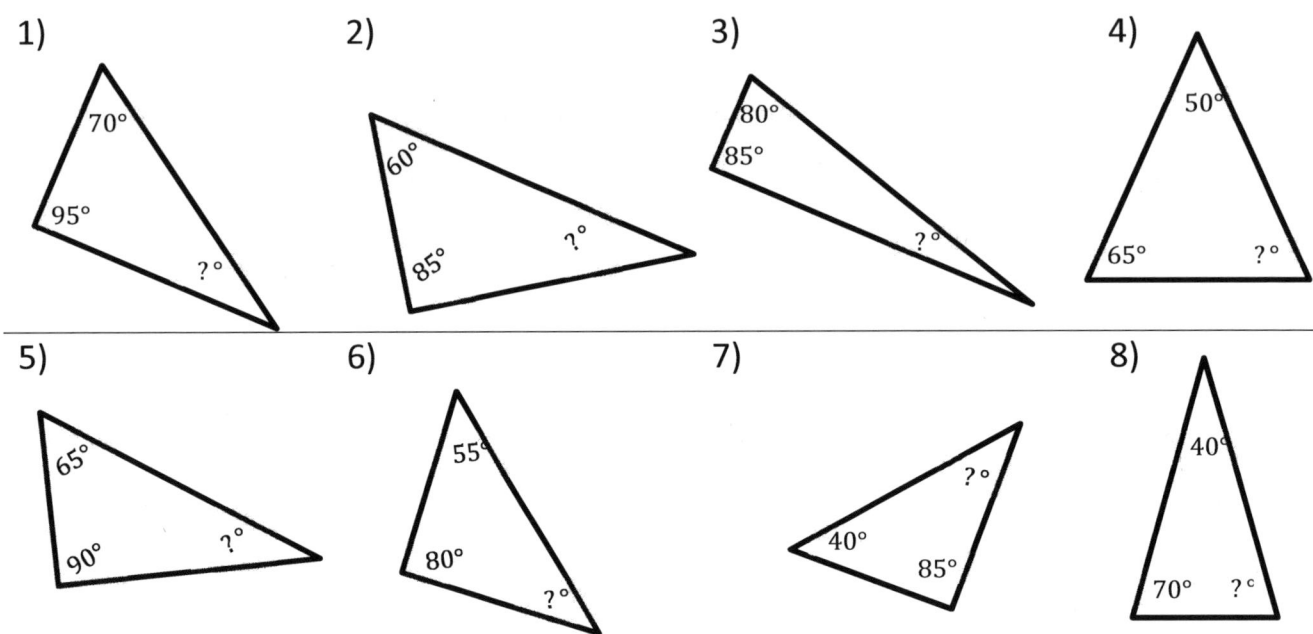

✎ **Find area of each triangle.**

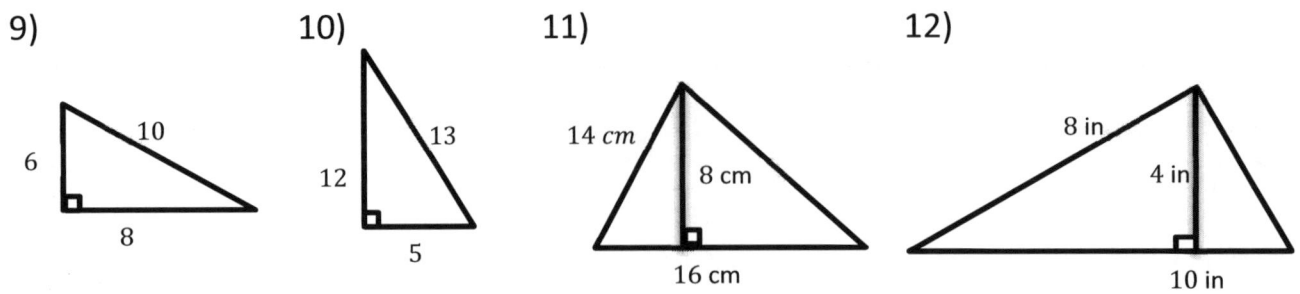

Polygons

✎ **Find the perimeter of each shape.**

1)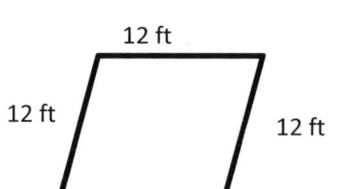

2)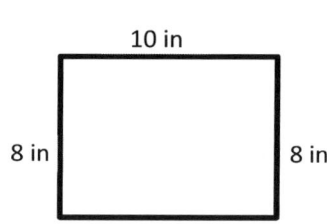

3)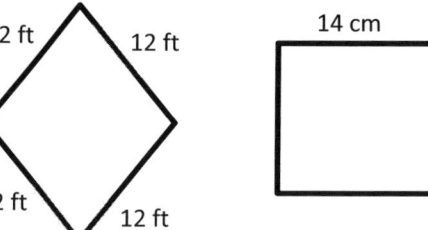

4) Square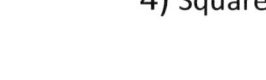

5) Regular hexagon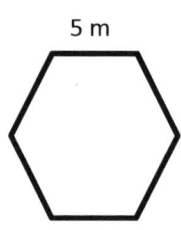

6)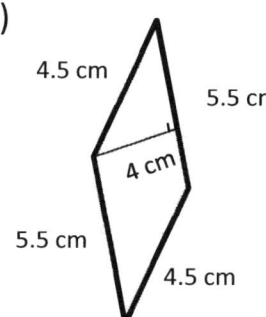

7) Parallelogram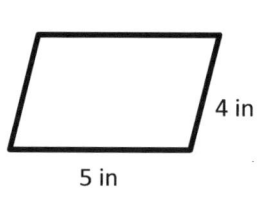

8) Square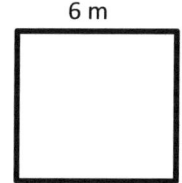

✎ **Find the area of each shape.**

9) Parallelogram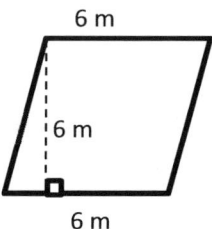

10) Rectangle

11) Rectangle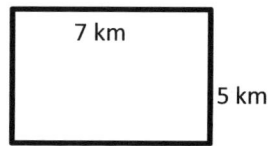

12) Square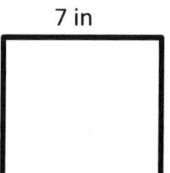

Trapezoids

✎ **Find the area of each trapezoid.**

1)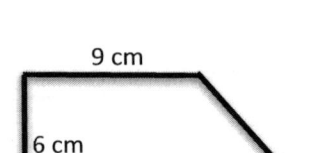

2)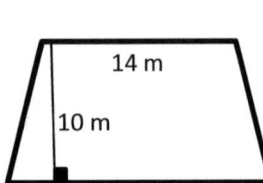

3)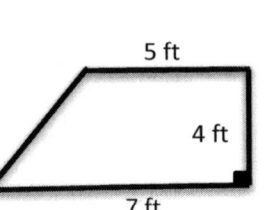

4)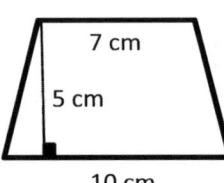

5)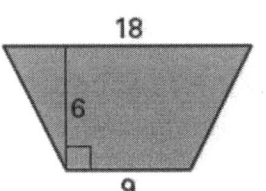

6)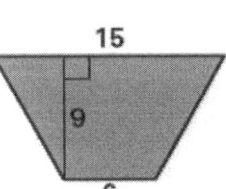

7)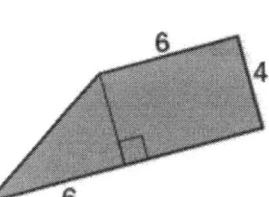

8)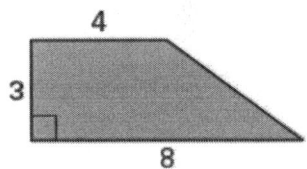

✎ **Solve.**

9) A trapezoid has an area of 60 cm² and its height is 6 cm and one base is 8 cm. What is the other base length? _____

10) If a trapezoid has an area of 65 ft² and the lengths of the bases are 12 ft and 14 ft, find the height. _____

11) If a trapezoid has an area of 180 m² and its height is 12 m and one base is 20 m, find the other base length. _____

12) The area of a trapezoid is 625 ft² and its height is 25 ft. If one base of the trapezoid is 15 ft, what is the other base length? _____

Circles

✎ **Find the area of each circle.** (π = 3.14)

1)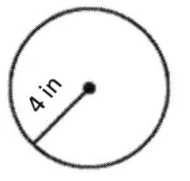
2)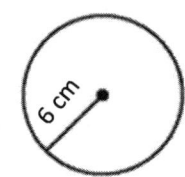
3)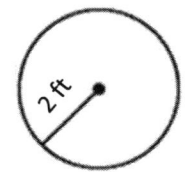
4)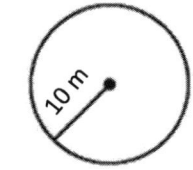
5)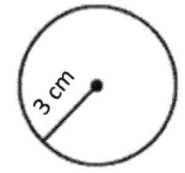
6)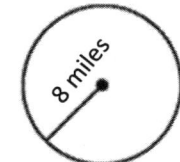

7)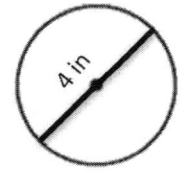
8)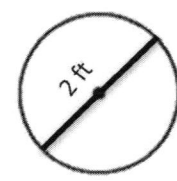
9)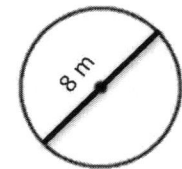
10)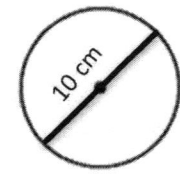
11)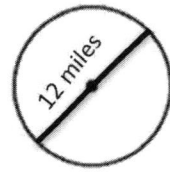
12)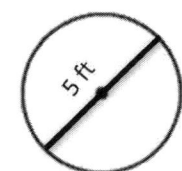

✎ **Complete the table below.** (π = 3.14)

	Radius	Diameter	Circumference	Area
Circle 1	4 inches	8 inches	25.12 inches	50.24 square inches
Circle 2		12 meters		
Circle 3				12.56 square ft
Circle 4			18.84 miles	
Circle 5		5 kilometers		
Circle 6	6 centimeters			
Circle 7		8 feet		
Circle 8				28.26 square meters
Circle 9			43.96 inches	
Circle 10	5 feet			

Cubes

✍ **Find the volume of each cube.**

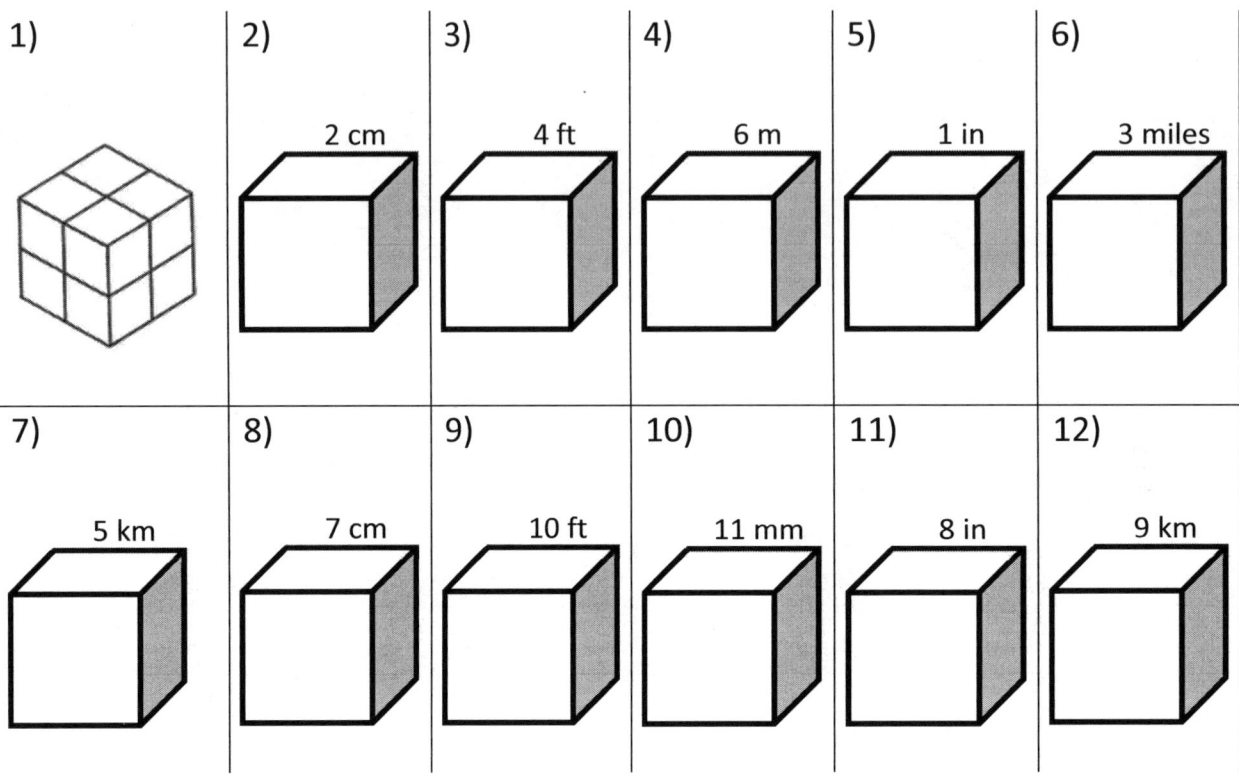

✍ **Find the surface area of each cube.**

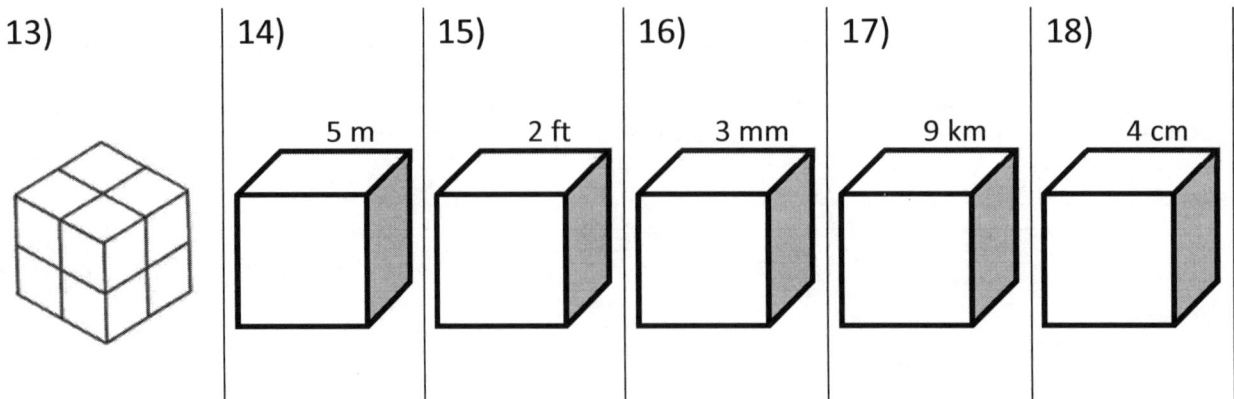

Rectangular Prism

✎ **Find the volume of each Rectangular Prism.**

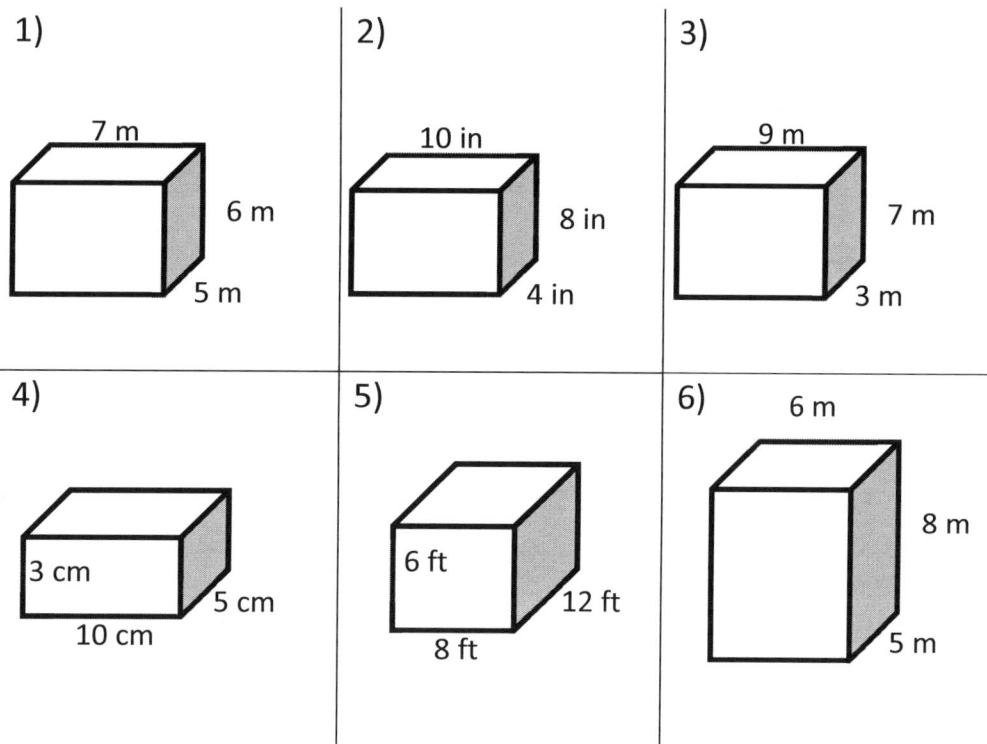

✎ **Find the surface area of each Rectangular Prism.**

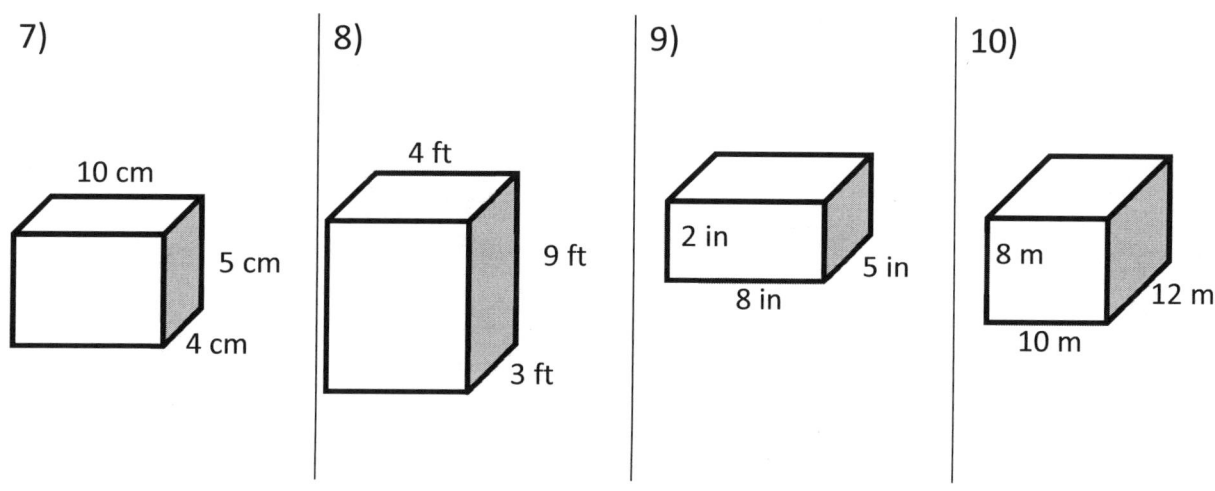

Cylinder

✎ **Find the volume of each Cylinder. Round your answer to the nearest tenth.** ($\pi = 3.14$)

1)
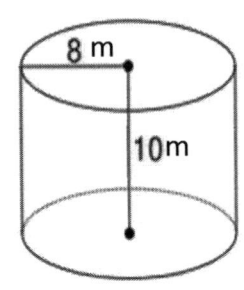

2)
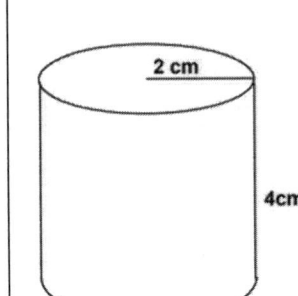

3)
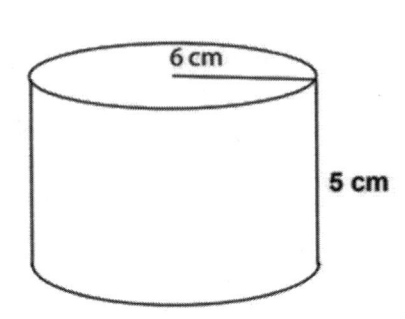

4)
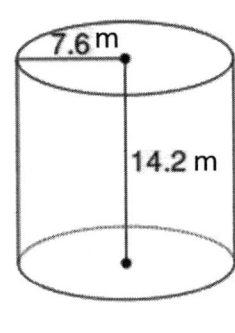

5)
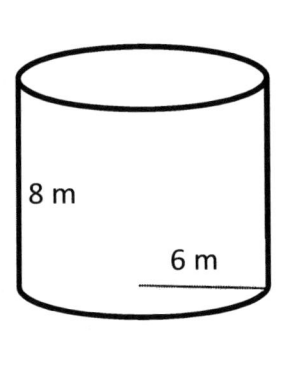

6)
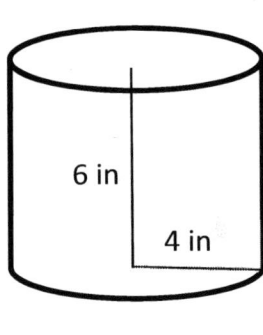

✎ **Find the surface area of each Cylinder.** ($\pi = 3.14$)

7)

8)

9)

10)

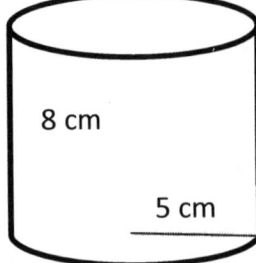
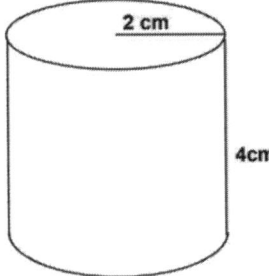
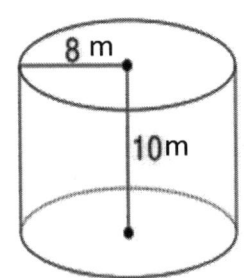

Pyramids and Cone

✎ **Find the volume of each Pyramid and Cone.** ($\pi = 3.14$)

1)

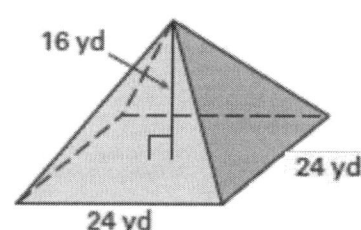

2)

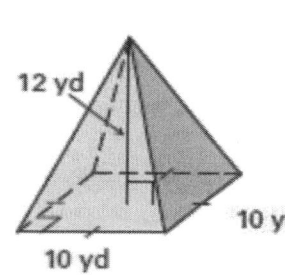

3)

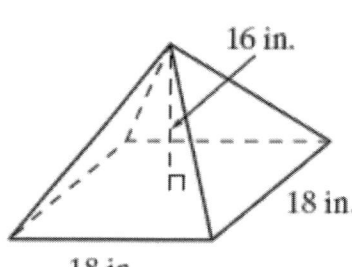

4)

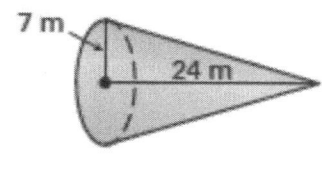

5)

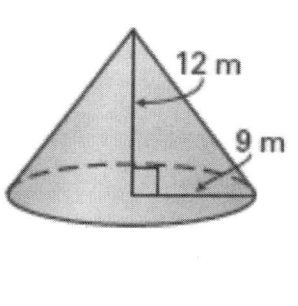

6)

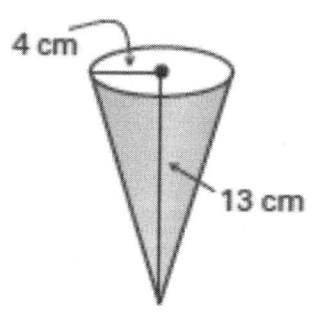

✎ **Find the surface area of each Pyramid and Cone.** ($\pi = 3.14$)

7)

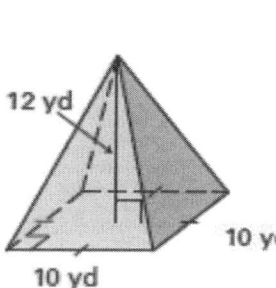

8)

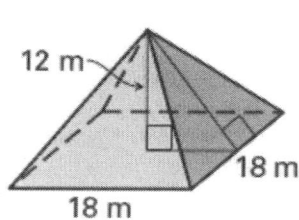

9)

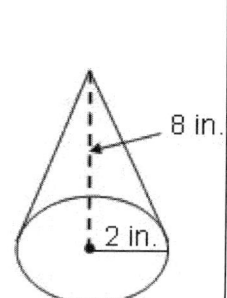

10)

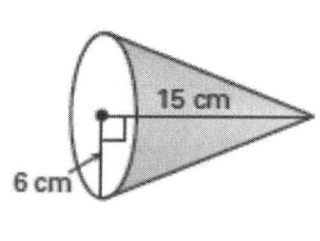

Answers of Worksheets – Chapter 12

Angles

1) 68°
2) 89°
3) 52°
4) 17°
5) 55°
6) 28°
7) 45°
8) 72°
9) 57°
10) 30°
11) 115°

Pythagorean Relationship

1) Yes
2) Yes
3) No
4) Yes
5) No
6) No
7) Yes
8) Yes
9) 5
10) 17
11) 15
12) 8
13) 5
14) 30
15) 30
16) 12

Triangles

1) 15°
2) 35°
3) 15°
4) 65°
5) 25°
6) 45°
7) 55°
8) 70°
9) 24 square unites
10) 30 square unites
11) 64 square unites
12) 20 square unites

Polygons

1) 48 ft
2) 36 in
3) 48 ft
4) 56 cm
5) 30 m
6) 20 cm
7) 18 in
8) 24 m
9) 36 m^2
10) 80 in^2
11) 35 km^2
12) 49 in^2

Trapezoids

1) 63 cm^2
2) 160 m^2
3) 24 ft^2
4) 42.5 cm^2
5) 81
6) 94.5
7) 36
8) 18
9) 12 cm
10) 5 ft
11) 10 m
12) 35 ft

Circles

1) 50.24 in^2
2) 113.04 cm^2
3) 12.56 ft^2
4) 314 m^2
5) 28.26 cm^2
6) 200.96 $miles^2$

7) $12.56\ in^2$
8) $3.14\ ft^2$
9) $50.24\ m^2$
10) $78.5\ cm^2$
11) $113.04\ miles^2$
12) $19.63\ ft^2$

	Radius	Diameter	Circumference	Area
Circle 1	4 inches	8 inches	25.12 inches	50.24 square inches
Circle 2	6 meters	12 meters	37.68 meters	113.04 meters
Circle 3	2 square ft	4 square ft	12.56 square ft	12.56 square ft
Circle 4	3 miles	6 miles	18.84 miles	28.26 miles
Circle 5	2.5 kilometers	5 kilometers	15.7 kilometers	19.63 kilometers
Circle 6	6 centimeters	12 centimeters	37.68 centimeters	113.04 centimeters
Circle 7	4 feet	8 feet	25.12 feet	50.24 feet
Circle 8	3 square meters	6 square meters	18.84 square meters	28.26 square meters
Circle 9	7 inches	14 inches	43.96 inches	153.86 inches
Circle 10	5 feet	10 feet	31.4 feet	78.5 feet

Cubes

1) 8
2) $8\ cm^3$
3) $64\ ft^3$
4) $216\ m^3$
5) $1\ in^3$
6) $27\ miles^3$
7) $125\ km^3$
8) $343\ cm^3$
9) $1,000\ ft^3$
10) $1,331\ mm^3$
11) $512\ in^3$
12) $729\ km^3$
13) 24
14) $150\ m^2$
15) $24\ ft^2$
16) $54\ mm^2$
17) $486\ km^2$
18) $96\ cm^2$

Rectangular Prism

1) $210\ m^3$
2) $320\ in^3$
3) $189\ m^3$
4) $150\ cm^3$
5) $576\ ft^3$
6) $240\ m^3$
7) $220\ cm^2$
8) $150\ ft^2$
9) $132\ in2$
10) $592\ m^2$

Cylinder

1) $2,009.6\ m^3$
2) $50.24\ cm^3$
3) $565.2\ cm^3$
4) $2,575.4\ m^3$
5) $904.3\ m^3$
6) $301.4\ in^3$
7) $251.2\ m^2$
8) $408.2\ cm^2$
9) $75.4\ cm^2$
10) $904.3\ m^2$

Pyramids and Cone

1) $3,072\ yd^3$
2) $400\ yd^3$
3) $1,728\ in^3$
4) $1,230.9\ m^3$
5) $1,017.9\ m^3$
6) $217.7\ cm^3$
7) $360\ yd^2$
8) $864\ m^2$
9) $64.34\ in^2$
10) $417.4\ cm^2$

Chapter 13:

Statistics and Probability

Topics that you'll practice in this chapter:

✓ Mean and Median

✓ Mode and Range

✓ Pie Graph

✓ Probability Problems

✓ Factorials

✓ Combinations and Permutations

Mathematics is no more computation than typing is literature.

– John Allen Paulos

Mean and Median

✎ **Find Mean and Median of the Given Data.**

1) 8, 12, 5, 3, 2

2) 3, 6, 3, 7, 4, 13

3) 13, 5, 1, 7, 9

4) 6, 4, 2, 7, 3, 2

5) 6, 5, 7, 5, 7, 1, 11

6) 6, 1, 4, 4, 9, 2, 19

7) 12, 4, 1, 5, 9, 7, 7, 19

8) 18, 9, 5, 4, 9, 6, 12

9) 28, 25, 15, 16, 32, 44, 71

10) 10, 5, 1, 5, 4, 5, 8, 10

11) 18, 15, 30, 64, 42, 11

12) 44, 33, 56, 78, 41, 84

✎ **Solve.**

13) In a javelin throw competition, five athletics score 56, 58, 63, 57 and 61 meters. What are their Mean and Median? _____

14) Eva went to shop and bought 3 apples, 5 peaches, 8 bananas, 1 pineapple and 3 melons. What are the Mean and Median of her purchase? _____

15) Bob has 12 black pen, 14 red pen, 15 green pens, 24 blue pens and 3 boxes of yellow pens. If the Mean and Median are 16 and 15 respectively, what is the number of yellow pens in each box? _____

Mode and Range

✎ **Find Mode and Rage of the Given Data.**

1) 8, 2, 5, 9, 1, 2

Mode: _____   Range: _____

2) 6, 6, 2, 3, 6, 3, 9, 12

Mode: _____   Range: _____

3) 4, 4, 3, 9, 7, 9, 4, 6, 4

Mode: _____   Range: _____

4) 12, 9, 2, 9, 3, 2, 9, 5

Mode: _____   Range: _____

5) 9, 5, 9, 5, 8, 9, 8

Mode: _____   Range: _____

6) 0, 1, 4, 10, 9, 2, 9, 1, 5, 1

Mode: _____   Range: _____

7) 6, 5, 6, 9, 7, 7, 5, 4, 3, 5

Mode: _____   Range: _____

8) 7, 5, 4, 9, 6, 7, 7, 5, 2

Mode: _____   Range: _____

9) 2, 2, 5, 6, 2, 4, 7, 6, 4, 9

Mode: _____   Range: _____

10) 7, 5, 2, 5, 4, 5, 8, 10

Mode: _____   Range: _____

11) 4, 1, 5, 2, 2, 12, 18, 2

Mode: _____   Range: _____

12) 6, 3, 5, 9, 6, 6, 3, 12

Mode: _____   Range: _____

✎ **Solve.**

13) A stationery sold 12 pencils, 36 red pens, 44 blue pens, 12 notebooks, 18 erasers, 34 rulers and 32 color pencils. What are the Mode and Range for the stationery sells?

Mode: _____   Range: _____

14) In an English test, eight students score 14, 13, 17, 11, 19, 20, 14 and 15. What are their Mode and Range? _____

15) What is the range of the first 6 even numbers greater than 11? _____

Pie Graph

The circle graph below shows all Jason's expenses for last month. Jason spent $300 on his bills last month.

Answer following questions based on the Pie graph.

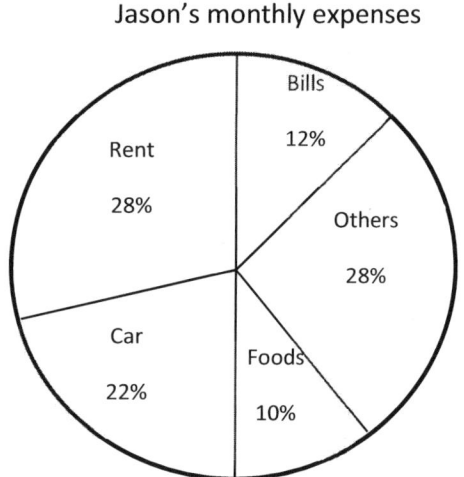

Jason's monthly expenses

1- How much did Jason spend on his car last month? _____

2- How much did Jason spend for foods last month? _____

3- How much did Jason spend on his rent last month? _____

4- What fraction is Jason's expenses for his bills and Car out of his total expenses last month? _____

5- How much was Jason's total expenses last month? _____

Probability Problems

✍ **Solve.**

1) A number is chosen at random from 1 to 10. Find the probability of selecting number 4 or smaller numbers. _____

2) Bag A contains 9 red marbles and 3 green marbles. Bag B contains 9 black marbles and 6 orange marbles. What is the probability of selecting a green marble at random from bag A? What is the probability of selecting a black marble at random from Bag B? _____ _____

3) A number is chosen at random from 1 to 50. What is the probability of selecting multiples of 10. _____

4) A card is chosen from a well-shuffled deck of 52 cards. What is the probability that the card will be a king OR a queen? _____

5) A number is chosen at random from 1 to 10. What is the probability of selecting a multiple of 3. _____

A spinner, numbered 1–8, is spun once. What is the probability of spinning ...

6) an EVEN number? _____   7) a multiple of 3? _____

8) a PRIME number? _____   9) number 9? _____

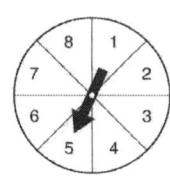

Factorials

✎ **Determine the value for each expression.**

1) $3! + 2! =$

2) $3! + 6! =$

3) $(3!)^2 =$

4) $5! + 4! =$

5) $4! - 5! + 4 =$

6) $2! \times 5 - 12 =$

7) $(2! + 1!)^3 =$

8) $(3! + 0!)^3 =$

9) $(2!\,0!)^4 - 1 =$

10) $\dfrac{7!}{4!} =$

11) $\dfrac{9!}{6!} =$

12) $\dfrac{8!}{5!} =$

13) $\dfrac{7!}{5!} =$

14) $\dfrac{20!}{18!} =$

15) $\dfrac{10!}{8!} =$

16) $\dfrac{(5+1!)^3}{3!} =$

17) $\dfrac{25!}{20!} =$

18) $\dfrac{22!}{18!\,5!} =$

19) $\dfrac{10!}{8!\,2!} =$

20) $\dfrac{100!}{97!} =$

21) $\dfrac{14!}{10!\,4!} =$

22) $\dfrac{14!}{9!\,3!} =$

23) $\dfrac{55!}{53!} =$

24) $\dfrac{(2 \cdot 3)!}{3!} =$

25) $\dfrac{4!(9n-1)!}{(9n)!} =$

26) $\dfrac{n(3n+8)!}{(3n+9)!} =$

27) $\dfrac{(n-2)!(n-1)}{(n+1)!} =$

Combinations and Permutations

✎ **Calculate the value of each.**

1) 4! = ____
2) 4! × 3! = ____
3) 5! = ____
4) 6! + 3! = ____
5) 7! = ____
6) 8! = ____
7) 4! + 4! = ____
8) 4! − 3! = ____

✎ **Solve each word problems.**

9) Susan is baking cookies. She uses sugar, flour, butter, and eggs. How many different orders of ingredients can she try? _____

10) Jason is planning for his vacation. He wants to go to museum, watch a movie, go to the beach, and play volleyball. How many different ways of ordering are there for him? _____

11) How many 5-digit numbers can be named using the digits 1, 2, 3, 4, and 5 without repetition? _____

12) In how many ways can 5 boys be arranDAT in a straight line? _____

13) In how many ways can 4 athletes be arranDAT in a straight line? _____

14) A professor is going to arrange her 7 students in a straight line. In how many ways can she do this? _____

15) How many code symbols can be formed with the letters for the word WHITE? _____

16) In how many ways a team of 8 basketball players can to choose a captain and co-captain? _____

Answers of Worksheets – Chapter 13

Mean and Median

1) Mean: 6, Median: 5
2) Mean: 6, Median: 5
3) Mean: 7, Median: 7
4) Mean: 4, Median: 3.5
5) Mean: 6, Median: 6

6) Mean: 8, Median: 4
7) Mean: 8, Median: 7
8) Mean: 9, Median: 9
9) Mean: 33, Median: 28
10) Mean: 6, Median: 5

11) Mean: 30, Median: 24
12) Mean: 56, Median: 50
13) Mean: 59, Median: 58
14) Mean: 4, Median: 3
15) 5

Mode and Range

1) Mode: 2, Range: 8
2) Mode: 6, Range: 10
3) Mode: 4, Range: 6
4) Mode: 9, Range: 10
5) Mode: 9, Range: 4

6) Mode: 1, Range: 10
7) Mode: 5, Range: 6
8) Mode: 7, Range: 7
9) Mode: 2, Range: 7
10) Mode: 5, Range: 8

11) Mode: 2, Range: 17
12) Mode: 6, Range: 9
13) Mode: 12, Range: 32
14) Mode: 14, Range: 9
15) 10

Pie Graph

1) $550
2) $250
3) $700

4) $\frac{17}{50}$
5) $2,500

Probability Problems

1) $\frac{2}{5}$
2) $\frac{1}{4}, \frac{3}{5}$
3) $\frac{1}{5}$

4) $\frac{2}{13}$
5) $\frac{3}{10}$
6) $\frac{1}{2}$

7) $\frac{1}{4}$
8) $\frac{1}{2}$
9) 0

Factorials

1) 8
2) 726
3) 36
4) 144

5) −92
6) −2
7) 27
8) 125

9) 15
10) 210
11) 504
12) 336

13) 42
14) 380
15) 90
16) 36
17) 6,375,600
18) 1,463
19) 45
20) 970,200
21) 1,001
22) 40,040
23) 2,970
24) 120
25) $\dfrac{8}{3n}$
26) $\dfrac{n}{3(n+3)}$
27) $\dfrac{1}{n(n+1)}$

Combinations and Permutations

1) 24
2) 144
3) 120
4) 726
5) 5,040
6) 40,320
7) 48
8) 18
9) 24
10) 24
11) 120
12) 120
13) 24
14) 5,040
15) 120
16) 56

Chapter 14:

Trigonometric Functions

Topics that you'll practice in this chapter:

- ✓ Trig ratios of General Angles
- ✓ Sketch Each Angle in Standard Position
- ✓ Finding Co–Terminal Angles and Reference Angles
- ✓ Angles in Radians
- ✓ Angles in Degrees
- ✓ Evaluating Each Trigonometric Expression
- ✓ Missing Sides and Angles of a Right Triangle
- ✓ Arc Length and Sector Area

Mathematics is like checkers in being suitable for the young, not too difficult, amusing, and without peril to the state. — Plato

Trig ratios of General Angles

✎ **Evaluate.**

1) $\sin -60° = $ _____

2) $\sin 150° = $ _____

3) $\cos 315° = $ _____

4) $\cos 180° = $ _____

5) $\sin 120° = $ _____

6) $\sin -330° = $ _____

7) $\tan -90° = $ _____

8) $\cot 90° = $ _____

9) $\tan 270° = $ _____

10) $\cot 150° = $ _____

11) $\sec 120° = $ _____

12) $\csc -360° = $ _____

13) $\cot -270° = $ _____

14) $\sec 90° = $ _____

15) $\cos -90° = $ _____

16) $\sec 60° = $ _____

17) $\csc 480° = $ _____

18) $\cot -135° = $ _____

✎ **Find the exact value of each trigonometric function. Some may be undefined.**

19) $\sec \pi = $ _____

20) $\tan -\frac{3\pi}{2} = $ _____

21) $\cos \frac{11\pi}{6} = $ _____

22) $\cot \frac{5\pi}{3} = $ _____

23) $\sec -\frac{3\pi}{4} = $ _____

24) $\sec \frac{\pi}{3} = $ _____

25) $\csc \frac{5\pi}{6} = $ _____

26) $\cot \frac{4\pi}{3} = $ _____

27) $\csc -\frac{3\pi}{4} = $ _____

28) $\cot \frac{2\pi}{3} = $ _____

Sketch Each Angle in Standard Position

✎ **Draw each angle with the given measure in standard position.**

1) $-120°$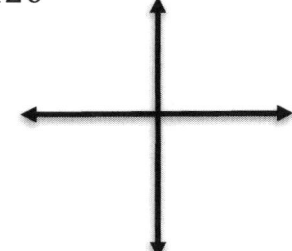

2) $440°$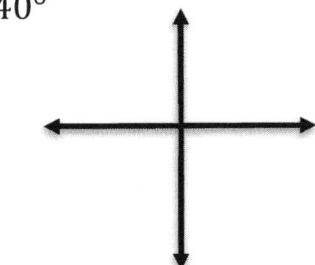

3) $-\dfrac{10\pi}{3}$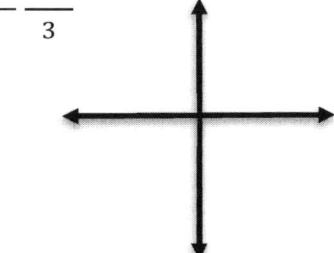

4) $280°$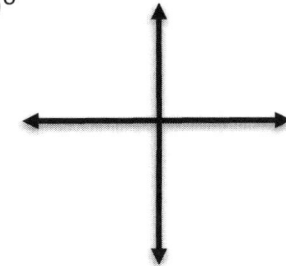

5) $710°$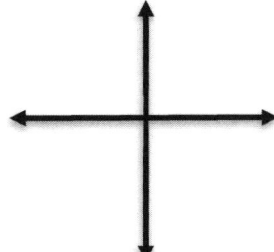

6) $\dfrac{11\pi}{6}$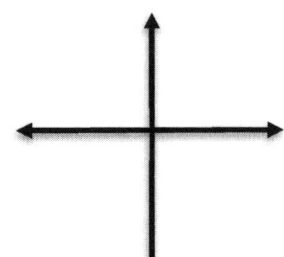

Angles and Angle Measure

✎ **Convert each degree measure into radians.**

1) $-140° =$ _____

2) $320° =$ _____

3) $210° =$ _____

4) $780° =$ _____

5) $-190° =$ _____

6) $345° =$ _____

7) $-150° =$ _____

8) $420° =$ _____

9) $300° =$ _____

10) $-60° =$ _____

11) $315° =$ _____

12) $600° =$ _____

13) $-720° =$ _____

14) $-160° =$ _____

15) $-210° =$ _____

16) $960° =$ _____

17) $-30° =$ _____

18) $660° =$ _____

19) $-240° =$ _____

20) $840° =$ _____

21) $1,200° =$ _____

✎ **Convert each radian measure into degrees.**

22) $\frac{\pi}{30} =$

23) $\frac{4\pi}{5} =$

24) $\frac{7\pi}{18} =$

25) $\frac{\pi}{5} =$

26) $-\frac{5\pi}{4} =$

27) $\frac{14\pi}{3} =$

28) $-\frac{16\pi}{3} =$

29) $-\frac{3\pi}{5} =$

30) $\frac{11\pi}{6} =$

31) $\frac{5\pi}{9} =$

32) $-\frac{\pi}{3} =$

33) $\frac{13\pi}{6} =$

34) $\frac{9\pi}{4} =$

35) $\frac{21}{4} =$

36) $-\frac{4\pi}{15} =$

37) $\frac{14}{3} =$

38) $-\frac{41\pi}{12} =$

39) $-\frac{17}{9} =$

Evaluating Trigonometric Functions

✍ **Find the exact value of each trigonometric function.**

1) $\cos 225° =$ _____

2) $\tan \dfrac{7\pi}{6} =$

3) $\tan -\dfrac{\pi}{6} =$ _____

4) $\cot -\dfrac{7\pi}{6} =$ _____

5) $\cos -\dfrac{\pi}{4} =$ _____

6) $\cos -480° =$ _____

7) $\sin 690° =$ _____

8) $\tan 420° =$ _____

9) $\cot -495° =$ _____

10) $\tan 405° =$ _____

11) $\cot 390° =$ _____

12) $\cos -300° =$ _____

13) $\cot -210° =$ _____

✍ **Use the given point on the terminal side of angle θ to find the value of the trigonometric function indicated.**

14) $\sin \theta;\ (-6, 4)$

15) $\cos \theta;\ (2, -2)$

16) $\cot \theta;\ (-7, \sqrt{15})$

17) $\cos \theta;\ (-5, -12)$

18) $\sin \theta;\ (-\sqrt{7}, 3)$

19) $\tan \theta;\ (-11, -2)$

Missing Sides and Angles of a Right Triangle

✎ **Find the value of each trigonometric ratio as fractions in their simplest form.**

1) $\tan A$

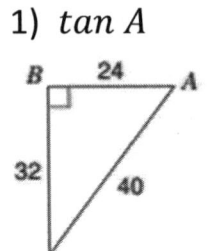

2) $\sin x$

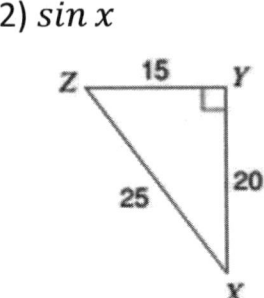

✎ **Find the missing sides. Round answers to the nearest tenth.**

3)

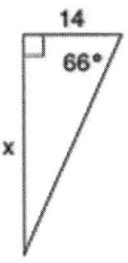

4)

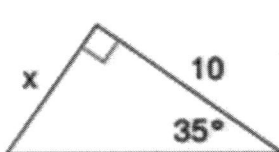

5)

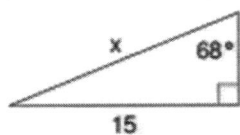

6)

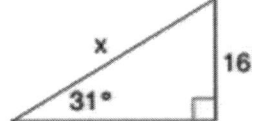

Arc Length and Sector Area

✎ **Find the length of each arc. Round your answers to the nearest tenth.**

   (π = 3.14)

1) $r = 28$ cm, $\theta = 45°$

2) $r = 15$ ft, $\theta = 95°$

3) $r = 22$ ft, $\theta = 60°$

4) $r = 12$ m, $\theta = 85°$

✎ **Find area of each sector. Do not round. Round your answers to the nearest tenth.** *(π = 3.14)*

5)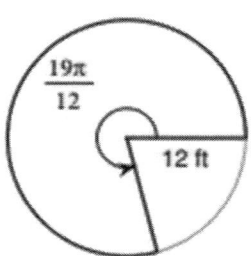

7)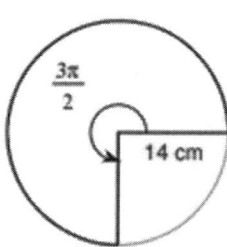

6)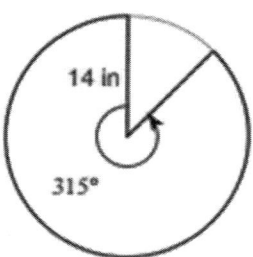

8)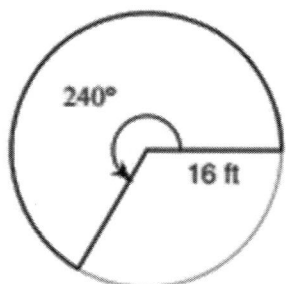

Answers of Worksheets – Chapter 14

Trig Ratios of General Angles

1) $-\frac{\sqrt{3}}{2}$

2) $\frac{1}{2}$

3) $\frac{\sqrt{2}}{2}$

4) -1

5) $\frac{\sqrt{3}}{2}$

6) $\frac{1}{2}$

7) Undefined

8) 0

9) Undefined

10) $-\sqrt{3}$

11) -2

12) 1

13) 0

14) Undefined

15) 0

16) 2

17) $\frac{2\sqrt{3}}{3}$

18) 1

19) -1

20) Undefined

21) $\frac{\sqrt{3}}{2}$

22) $-\frac{\sqrt{3}}{3}$

23) $-\sqrt{2}$

24) 2

25) 2

26) $\frac{\sqrt{3}}{3}$

27) $-\sqrt{2}$

28) $-\frac{\sqrt{3}}{3}$

Sketch Each Angle in Standard Position

1) $-120°$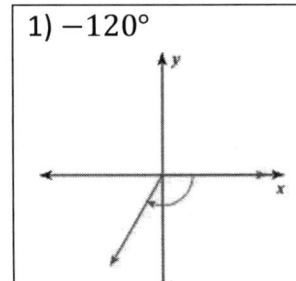

2) $440°$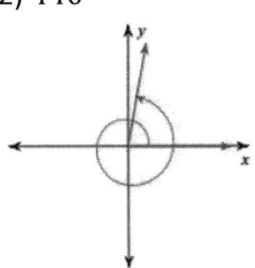

3) $-\frac{10\pi}{3}$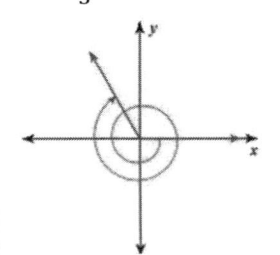

4) $280°$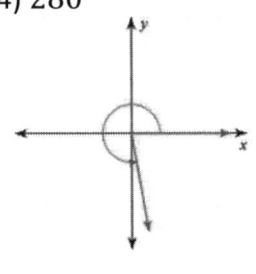

5) $710°$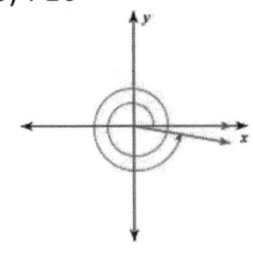

6) $\frac{11\pi}{6}$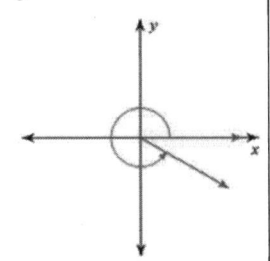

Angles and Angle Measure

1) $-\frac{7\pi}{9}$
2) $\frac{16\pi}{9}$
3) $\frac{7\pi}{6}$
4) $\frac{13}{3}$
5) $-\frac{19}{18}$
6) $\frac{23\pi}{12}$
7) $-\frac{5\pi}{6}$
8) $\frac{7\pi}{3}$
9) $\frac{5\pi}{3}$
10) $-\frac{\pi}{3}$
11) $\frac{7\pi}{4}$
12) $\frac{10}{3}$
13) -4π
14) $-\frac{8\pi}{9}$
15) $-\frac{7\pi}{6}$
16) $\frac{16}{3}$
17) $-\frac{\pi}{6}$
18) $\frac{11}{3}$
19) $-\frac{4\pi}{3}$
20) $\frac{14\pi}{3}$
21) $\frac{20}{3}$
22) $6°$
23) $144°$
24) $70°$
25) $36°$
26) $-225°$
27) $840°$
28) $-960°$
29) $-108°$
30) $330°$
31) $100°$
32) $-60°$
33) $390°$
34) $405°$
35) $945°$
36) $-48°$
37) $840°$
38) $-615°$
39) $-340°$

Evaluating Each Trigonometric Expression

1) $-\frac{\sqrt{2}}{2}$
2) $\frac{\sqrt{3}}{3}$
3) $-\frac{\sqrt{3}}{3}$
4) $-\sqrt{3}$
5) $\frac{\sqrt{2}}{2}$
6) $-\frac{1}{2}$
7) $-\frac{1}{2}$
8) $\sqrt{3}$
9) 1
10) 1
11) $\sqrt{3}$
12) $\frac{1}{2}$
13) $-\sqrt{3}$
14) $\frac{2\sqrt{13}}{13}$
15) $\sqrt{2}$
16) $-\frac{7\sqrt{15}}{15}$
17) $-\frac{5}{13}$
18) $\frac{3}{4}$
19) $\frac{2}{11}$

Missing Sides and Angles of a Right Triangle

159

1) $\frac{4}{3}$
2) $\frac{3}{5}$
3) 31.4
4) 7.0
5) 16.2
6) 31.1

Arc Length and Sector Area

1) 22 cm
2) 24.9 ft
3) 23 ft
4) 17.8 m
5) 358 ft^2
6) 538.5 in^2
7) 461.6 cm^2
8) 535.9 ft^2

DAT Test Review

The Dental Admission Test (also known as the DAT) is a standardized test designed by the American Dental Association (ADA) to measure the general academic skills and perceptual ability of dental school applicants.

The DAT is comprised of multiple-choice test items consisting of four sections:

- ✓ Survey of the Natural Sciences
- ✓ Perceptual Ability
- ✓ Reading Comprehension
- ✓ Quantitative Reasoning

The Quantitative Reasoning section of the DAT measures applicants' Quantitative Reasoning skills that will be required in dental schools. There are 40 multiple-choice questions test takers have 45 minutes to complete this section. A basic four function calculator on the computer screen will be available on this section.

In this book, we have reviewed Quantitative Reasoning topics being tested on the DAT. In this section, there are two complete DAT Quantitative Reasoning Tests. Take these tests to see what score you will be able to receive on a real DAT test.

Good luck!

DAT Quantitative Reasoning Practice Tests

Time to Test

Time to refine your quantitative reasoning skill with a practice test

In this section, there are two complete DAT Quantitative Reasoning practice tests. Take these tests to simulate the test day experience. After you've finished, score your tests using the answer keys.

Before You Start

- You'll need a pencil, a calculator and a timer to take the test.
- For each question, there are five possible answers. Choose which one is best.
- It's okay to guess. There is no penalty for wrong answers.
- Use the answer sheet provided to record your answers.
- After you've finished the test, review the answer key to see where you went wrong.

Good Luck!

Mathematics is like love; a simple idea, but it can get complicated.

DAT Practice Tests Answer Sheet

Remove (or photocopy) this answer sheet and use it to complete the practice tests.

DAT Quantitative Reasoning Practice Tests Answer Sheet

DAT Practice Test 1

#		#		#	
1	Ⓐ Ⓑ Ⓒ Ⓓ Ⓔ	16	Ⓐ Ⓑ Ⓒ Ⓓ Ⓔ	31	Ⓐ Ⓑ Ⓒ Ⓓ Ⓔ
2	Ⓐ Ⓑ Ⓒ Ⓓ Ⓔ	17	Ⓐ Ⓑ Ⓒ Ⓓ Ⓔ	32	Ⓐ Ⓑ Ⓒ Ⓓ Ⓔ
3	Ⓐ Ⓑ Ⓒ Ⓓ Ⓔ	18	Ⓐ Ⓑ Ⓒ Ⓓ Ⓔ	33	Ⓐ Ⓑ Ⓒ Ⓓ Ⓔ
4	Ⓐ Ⓑ Ⓒ Ⓓ Ⓔ	19	Ⓐ Ⓑ Ⓒ Ⓓ Ⓔ	34	Ⓐ Ⓑ Ⓒ Ⓓ Ⓔ
5	Ⓐ Ⓑ Ⓒ Ⓓ Ⓔ	20	Ⓐ Ⓑ Ⓒ Ⓓ Ⓔ	35	Ⓐ Ⓑ Ⓒ Ⓓ Ⓔ
6	Ⓐ Ⓑ Ⓒ Ⓓ Ⓔ	21	Ⓐ Ⓑ Ⓒ Ⓓ Ⓔ	36	Ⓐ Ⓑ Ⓒ Ⓓ Ⓔ
7	Ⓐ Ⓑ Ⓒ Ⓓ Ⓔ	22	Ⓐ Ⓑ Ⓒ Ⓓ Ⓔ	37	Ⓐ Ⓑ Ⓒ Ⓓ Ⓔ
8	Ⓐ Ⓑ Ⓒ Ⓓ Ⓔ	23	Ⓐ Ⓑ Ⓒ Ⓓ Ⓔ	38	Ⓐ Ⓑ Ⓒ Ⓓ Ⓔ
9	Ⓐ Ⓑ Ⓒ Ⓓ Ⓔ	24	Ⓐ Ⓑ Ⓒ Ⓓ Ⓔ	39	Ⓐ Ⓑ Ⓒ Ⓓ Ⓔ
10	Ⓐ Ⓑ Ⓒ Ⓓ Ⓔ	25	Ⓐ Ⓑ Ⓒ Ⓓ Ⓔ	40	Ⓐ Ⓑ Ⓒ Ⓓ Ⓔ
11	Ⓐ Ⓑ Ⓒ Ⓓ Ⓔ	26	Ⓐ Ⓑ Ⓒ Ⓓ Ⓔ		
12	Ⓐ Ⓑ Ⓒ Ⓓ Ⓔ	27	Ⓐ Ⓑ Ⓒ Ⓓ Ⓔ		
13	Ⓐ Ⓑ Ⓒ Ⓓ Ⓔ	28	Ⓐ Ⓑ Ⓒ Ⓓ Ⓔ		
14	Ⓐ Ⓑ Ⓒ Ⓓ Ⓔ	29	Ⓐ Ⓑ Ⓒ Ⓓ Ⓔ		
15	Ⓐ Ⓑ Ⓒ Ⓓ Ⓔ	30	Ⓐ Ⓑ Ⓒ Ⓓ Ⓔ		

DAT Practice Test 2

#		#		#	
1	Ⓐ Ⓑ Ⓒ Ⓓ Ⓔ	16	Ⓐ Ⓑ Ⓒ Ⓓ Ⓔ	31	Ⓐ Ⓑ Ⓒ Ⓓ Ⓔ
2	Ⓐ Ⓑ Ⓒ Ⓓ Ⓔ	17	Ⓐ Ⓑ Ⓒ Ⓓ Ⓔ	32	Ⓐ Ⓑ Ⓒ Ⓓ Ⓔ
3	Ⓐ Ⓑ Ⓒ Ⓓ Ⓔ	18	Ⓐ Ⓑ Ⓒ Ⓓ Ⓔ	33	Ⓐ Ⓑ Ⓒ Ⓓ Ⓔ
4	Ⓐ Ⓑ Ⓒ Ⓓ Ⓔ	19	Ⓐ Ⓑ Ⓒ Ⓓ Ⓔ	34	Ⓐ Ⓑ Ⓒ Ⓓ Ⓔ
5	Ⓐ Ⓑ Ⓒ Ⓓ Ⓔ	20	Ⓐ Ⓑ Ⓒ Ⓓ Ⓔ	35	Ⓐ Ⓑ Ⓒ Ⓓ Ⓔ
6	Ⓐ Ⓑ Ⓒ Ⓓ Ⓔ	21	Ⓐ Ⓑ Ⓒ Ⓓ Ⓔ	36	Ⓐ Ⓑ Ⓒ Ⓓ Ⓔ
7	Ⓐ Ⓑ Ⓒ Ⓓ Ⓔ	22	Ⓐ Ⓑ Ⓒ Ⓓ Ⓔ	37	Ⓐ Ⓑ Ⓒ Ⓓ Ⓔ
8	Ⓐ Ⓑ Ⓒ Ⓓ Ⓔ	23	Ⓐ Ⓑ Ⓒ Ⓓ Ⓔ	38	Ⓐ Ⓑ Ⓒ Ⓓ Ⓔ
9	Ⓐ Ⓑ Ⓒ Ⓓ Ⓔ	24	Ⓐ Ⓑ Ⓒ Ⓓ Ⓔ	39	Ⓐ Ⓑ Ⓒ Ⓓ Ⓔ
10	Ⓐ Ⓑ Ⓒ Ⓓ Ⓔ	25	Ⓐ Ⓑ Ⓒ Ⓓ Ⓔ	40	Ⓐ Ⓑ Ⓒ Ⓓ Ⓔ
11	Ⓐ Ⓑ Ⓒ Ⓓ Ⓔ	26	Ⓐ Ⓑ Ⓒ Ⓓ Ⓔ		
12	Ⓐ Ⓑ Ⓒ Ⓓ Ⓔ	27	Ⓐ Ⓑ Ⓒ Ⓓ Ⓔ		
13	Ⓐ Ⓑ Ⓒ Ⓓ Ⓔ	28	Ⓐ Ⓑ Ⓒ Ⓓ Ⓔ		
14	Ⓐ Ⓑ Ⓒ Ⓓ Ⓔ	29	Ⓐ Ⓑ Ⓒ Ⓓ Ⓔ		
15	Ⓐ Ⓑ Ⓒ Ⓓ Ⓔ	30	Ⓐ Ⓑ Ⓒ Ⓓ Ⓔ		

DAT Quantitative Reasoning Practice Test 1

40 questions

Total time for this section: 45 Minutes

You may use a basic calculator on this test.

1) The marked price of a computer is D dollar. Its price decreased by 20% in January and later increased by 10 % in February. What is the final price of the computer in D dollar?

A. 0.80 D

B. 0.88 D

C. 0.90 D

D. 1.20 D

E. 1.40 D

2) The number 40.5 is 1,000 times greater than which of the following numbers?

A. 0.405

B. 0.0405

C. 0.0450

D. 0.00405

E. 0.000405

3) How many tiles of 8 cm^2 is needed to cover a floor of dimension 6 cm by 24 cm?

A. 6

B. 12

C. 18

D. 24

E. 36

4) What is the area of a square whose diagonal is 8 cm?

A. 16 cm²

B. 32 cm²

C. 36 cm²

D. 64 cm²

E. 128 cm²

5) What is the value of x in the following figure?

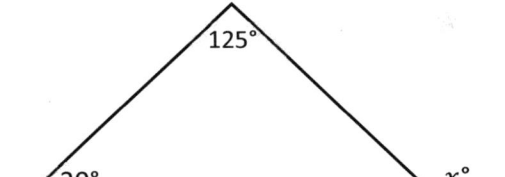

A. 150

B. 145

C. 125

D. 105

E. 95

6) Right triangle ABC is shown below. Which of the following is true for all possible values of angle A and B?

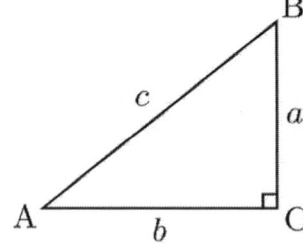

A. $\tan A = \tan B$

B. $\sin A = \cos B$

C. $\tan^2 A = \tan^2 B$

D. $\tan A = 1$

E. $\cot A = \sin B$

7) What is the value of y in the following system of equation?

$$3x - 4y = -20$$
$$-x + 2y = 10$$

A. -1

B. -2

C. 1

D. 4

E. 5

8) How long does a 420–miles trip take moving at 50 miles per hour (mph)?

A. 4 hours

B. 6 hours and 24 minutes

C. 8 hours and 24 minutes

D. 8 hours and 30 minutes

E. 10 hours and 30 minutes

9) From the figure, which of the following must be true? (figure not drawn to scale)

A. $y = z$

B. $y = 5x$

C. $y \geq x$

D. $y + 4x = z$

E. $y > x$

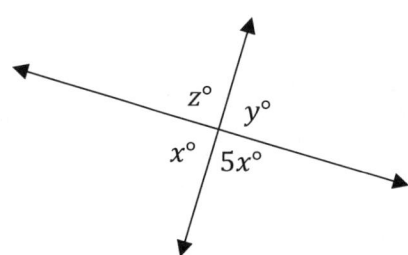

10) When 40% of 60 is added to 12% of 600, the resulting number is:

A. 24
B. 72
C. 96
D. 140
E. 180

11) A chemical solution contains 4% alcohol. If there is 24 ml of alcohol, what is the volume of the solution?

A. 240 ml
B. 480 ml
C. 600 ml
D. 1,200 ml
E. 2,400 ml

12) Which of the following points lies on the line $2x + 4y = 10$?

A. (2,1)
B. (−1,3)
C. (−2,2)
D. (2,2)
E. (2,8)

13) In the following figure, $ABCD$ is a rectangle, and E and F are points on AD and DC, respectively. The area of $\triangle BED$ is 16, and the area of $\triangle BDF$ is 18. What is the perimeter of the rectangle?

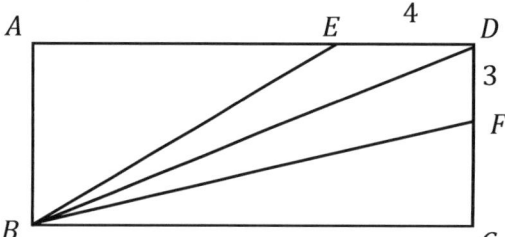

A. 20

B. 22

C. 32

D. 40

E. 44

14) What is the solution of the following inequality?

$$|x - 10| \leq 3$$

A. $x \geq 13 \ \cup \ x \leq 7$

B. $7 \leq x \leq 13$

C. $x \geq 13$

D. $x \leq 7$

E. Set of real numbers

15) A bag contains 18 balls: two green, five black, eight blue, a brown, a red and one white. If 17 balls are removed from the bag at random, what is the probability that a brown ball has been removed?

A. $\dfrac{1}{9}$

B. $\dfrac{1}{6}$

C. $\dfrac{16}{17}$

D. $\dfrac{17}{18}$

E. $\dfrac{1}{2}$

16) If a tree casts a 24–foot shadow at the same time that a 3 feet yardstick casts a 2–foot shadow, what is the height of the tree?

A. 24 ft

B. 28 ft

C. 36 ft

D. 48 ft

E. 52 ft

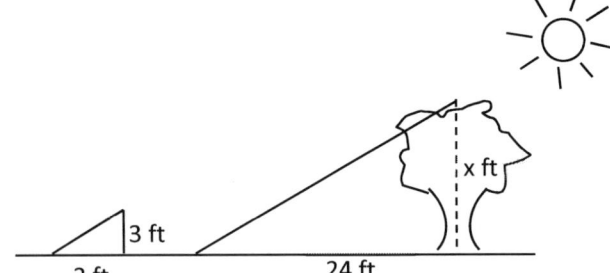

17) A ladder leans against a wall forming a 60° angle between the ground and the ladder. If the bottom of the ladder is 30 feet away from the wall, how long is the ladder?

A. 30 feet
B. 40 feet
C. 50 feet
D. 60 feet
E. 120 feet

18) If 40 % of a class are girls, and 25 % of girls play tennis, what percent of the class play tennis?

A. 10 %
B. 15%
C. 20 %
D. 40 %
E. 80 %

19) In five successive hours, a car travels 40 km, 45 km, 50 km, 35 km and 55 km. In the next five hours, it travels with an average speed of 50 km per hour. Find the total distance the car traveled in 10 hours.

A. 425 km
B. 450 km
C. 475 km
D. 500 km
E. 1,000 km

20) From last year, the price of gasoline has increased from $1.25 per gallon to $1.75 per gallon. The new price is what percent of the original price?

A. 72%

B. 120%

C. 140%

D. 160%

E. 180%

21) If $\frac{3x}{16} = \frac{x-1}{4}$, $x =$

A. $\frac{1}{4}$

B. $\frac{3}{4}$

C. 3

D. 4

E. $\frac{9}{4}$

22) If $\tan \theta = \frac{5}{12}$ and $\sin \theta > 0$, then $\cos \theta = ?$

A. $-\frac{5}{13}$

B. $\frac{12}{13}$

C. $\frac{13}{12}$

D. $-\frac{12}{13}$

E. 0

23) If 60% of x equal to 30% of 20, then what is the value of $(x+5)^2$?

A. 25.25

B. 26

C. 26.01

D. 2025

E. 225

24) In the xy-plane, the point $(4, 3)$ and $(3, 2)$ are on line A. Which of the following equations of lines is parallel to line A?

A. $y = 3x$

B. $y = 10$

C. $y = \frac{x}{2}$

D. $y = 2x$

E. $y = x$

25) When point A $(10, 3)$ is reflected over the y-axis to get the point B, what are the coordinates of point B?

A. $(10, 3)$

B. $(-10, -3)$

C. $(-10, 3)$

D. $(10, -3)$

E. $(0, 3)$

26) If the area of trapezoid is 100, what is the perimeter of the trapezoid?

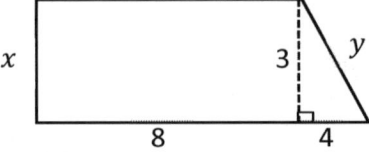

A. 25

B. 35

C. 45

D. 55

E. 65

27) A number is chosen at random from 1 to 25. Find the probability of not selecting a composite number.

A. $\dfrac{1}{25}$

B. 25

C. $\dfrac{2}{5}$

D. 1

E. 0

28) Removing which of the following numbers will change the average of the numbers to 6?

1, 4, 5, 8, 11, 12

A. 1

B. 4

C. 5

D. 11

E. 12

29) A rope weighs 600 grams per meter of length. What is the weight in kilograms of 12.2 meters of this rope? (1 kilograms = 1000 grams)

A. 0.0732

B. 0.732

C. 7.32

D. 7,320

E. 73,200

30) If $y = 4ab + 3b^3$, what is y when $a = 2$ and $b = 3$?

A. 24

B. 31

C. 36

D. 51

E. 105

31) If $f(x) = 5 + x$ and $g(x) = -x^2 - 1 - 2x$, then find $(g - f)(x)$?

A. $x^2 - 3x - 6$

B. $x^2 - 3x + 6$

C. $-x^2 - 3x + 6$

D. $-x^2 - 3x - 6$

E. $-x^2 + 3x - 6$

32) If $f(x) = 2x^3 + 5x^2 + 2x$ and $g(x) = -2$, what is the value of $f(g(x))$?

A. 36

B. 32

C. 24

D. 4

E. 0

33) In the following equation when z is divided by 3, what is the effect on x?

$$x = \frac{8y + \frac{r}{r+1}}{\frac{6}{z}}$$

A. x is divided by 2

B. x is divided by 3

C. x does not change

D. x is multiplied by 3

E. x is multiplied by 2

34) A boat sails 40 miles south and then 30 miles east. How far is the boat from its start point?

A. 45 miles

B. 50 miles

C. 60 miles

D. 70 miles

E. 80 miles

35) x is y% of what number?

A. $\dfrac{100x}{y}$

B. $\dfrac{100y}{x}$

C. $\dfrac{x}{100y}$

D. $\dfrac{y}{100x}$

E. $\dfrac{xy}{100}$

36) If cotangent of an angel β is 1, then the tangent of angle β is

A. -1

B. 0

C. 1

D. 2

E. 3

37) 6 liters of water are poured into an aquarium that's 15cm long, 5cm wide, and 60cm high. How many cm will the water level in the aquarium rise due to this added water? (1 liter of water = 1000 cm³)

A. 80

B. 40

C. 20

D. 10

E. 5

38) If a box contains red and blue balls in ratio of 2 : 3, how many red balls are there if 90 blue balls are in the box?

A. 90

B. 60

C. 30

D. 10

E. 8

39) If $|a| < 1$, then which of the following is true? ($b > 0$)?

   I. $-b < ba < b$

   II. $-a < a^2 < a \quad if \quad a < 0$

   III. $-5 < 2a - 3 < -1$

A. I only

B. II only

C. I and III only

D. III only

E. I, II and III

40) What is the surface area of the cylinder below?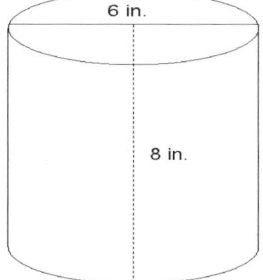

A. 48 π in²

B. 57 π in²

C. 66 π in²

D. 288 π in²

E. 400 π in²

The End of Practice Test 1

DAT Quantitative Reasoning

Practice Test 2

40 questions

Total time for this section: 45 Minutes

You may use a basic calculator on this test.

1) If $f(x) = 3x - 1$ and $g(x) = x^2 - x$, then find $(\frac{f}{g})(x)$.

   A. $\frac{3x-1}{x^2-x}$

   B. $\frac{x-1}{x^2-x}$

   C. $\frac{x-1}{x^2-1}$

   D. $\frac{3x+1}{x^2+x}$

   E. $\frac{x^2-x}{3x-1}$

2) In the standard (x, y) coordinate plane, which of the following lines contains the points $(3, -5)$ and $(8, 15)$?

   A. $y = 4x - 17$

   B. $y = \frac{1}{4}x + 13$

   C. $y = -4x + 7$

   D. $y = -\frac{1}{4}x + 17$

   E. $y = 2x - 11$

3) A bank is offering 3.5% simple interest on a savings account. If you deposit $12,000, how much interest will you earn in two years?

   A. $420

   B. $840

   C. $4,200

   D. $8,400

   E. $9,600

4) If the ratio of home fans to visiting fans in a crowd is 3:2 and all 25,000 seats in a stadium are filled, how many visiting fans are in attendance?

   A. 100,000
   B. 100
   C. 1,000
   D. 10
   E. 10,000

5) If the interior angles of a quadrilateral are in the ratio 1:2:2:5, what is the measure of the largest angle?

   A. 36°
   B. 72°
   C. 108°
   D. 144°
   E. 180°

6) If the area of a circle is 64 square meters, what is its diameter?

   A. 8π
   B. $8\sqrt{\pi}$
   C. $\frac{8\sqrt{\pi}}{\pi}$
   D. $\frac{8}{\pi}$
   E. $64\pi^2$

7) The length of a rectangle is $\frac{5}{4}$ times its width. If the width is 16, what is the perimeter of this rectangle?

   A. 36
   B. 48
   C. 72
   D. 144
   E. 180

8) In the figure below, line A is parallel to line B. What is the value of angle x?

   A. 35 degree
   B. 45 degree
   C. 90 degree
   D. 100 degree
   E. 145 degree

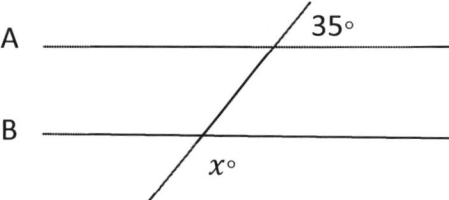

9) Last week 24,000 fans attended a football match. This week three times as many bought tickets, but one sixth of them cancelled their tickets. How many are attending this week?

   A. 60,000
   B. 72,000
   C. 48,000
   D. 54,000
   E. 84,000

10) If $\sin A = \frac{1}{3}$ in a right triangle and the angle A is an acute angle, then what is $\cos A$?

   A. $\frac{\sqrt{8}}{3}$

   B. $\frac{2}{3}$

   C. $\frac{\sqrt{3}}{8}$

   D. $\frac{\sqrt{8}}{9}$

   E. $\frac{9}{\sqrt{8}}$

11) If $(x-2)^2 + 1 > 3x - 1$, then x can equal which of the following?

   A. 1
   B. 6
   C. 8
   D. 3
   E. 4

12) If 150% of a number is 75, then what is 90% of that number?

   A. 45
   B. 50
   C. 70
   D. 85
   E. 90

13) The width of a box is one third of its length. The height of the box is one third of its width. If the length of the box is 27 cm, what is the volume of the box?

A. 81 cm³

B. 162 cm³

C. 243 cm³

D. 729 cm³

E. 1880 cm³

14) What is the solution of the following inequality?

$$|x - 2| \geq 3$$

A. $x \geq 5 \cup x \leq -1$

B. $-1 \leq x \leq 5$

C. $x \geq 5$

D. $x \leq -1$

E. Set of real numbers

15) If $\tan x = \frac{8}{15}$, then $\sin x =$

A. $\frac{1}{2}$

B. $\frac{8}{17}$

C. $\frac{15}{17}$

D. $\frac{7}{15}$

E. It cannot be determined from the information given.

16) In the following figure, $ABCD$ is a rectangle. If $a = \sqrt{3}$, and $b = 2a$, find the area of the shaded region. (the shaded region is a trapezoid)

A. 4

B. 2

C. $\sqrt{3}$

D. $2\sqrt{3}$

E. $4\sqrt{3}$

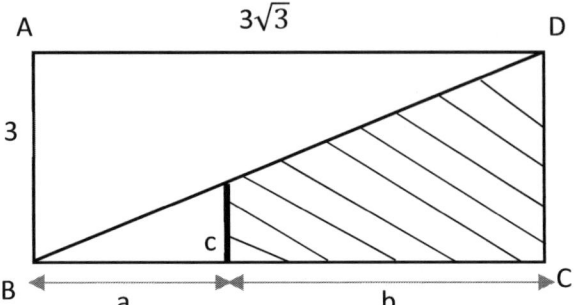

17) Convert 670,000 to scientific notation.

A. 6.70×1000

B. 6.70×10^{-5}

C. 6.7×100

D. 6.7×10^5

E. 6.7×10^4

18) In two successive years, the population of a town is increased by 15% and 20%. What percent of the population is increased after two years?

A. 32%

B. 35%

C. 38%

D. 68%

E. 70%

19) $(x^6)^{\frac{5}{8}}$ equal to?

A. $x^{\frac{15}{4}}$

B. $x^{\frac{53}{8}}$

C. $x^{\frac{4}{15}}$

D. $x^{\frac{8}{53}}$

E. $x^{\frac{5}{48}}$

20) If one angle of a right triangle measures 60°, what is the sine of the other acute angle?

A. $\frac{1}{2}$

B. $\frac{\sqrt{2}}{2}$

C. $\frac{\sqrt{3}}{2}$

D. 1

E. $\sqrt{3}$

21) In the following figure, what is the perimeter of $\triangle ABC$ if the area of $\triangle ADC$ is 15?

A. 37.5

B. 21

C. 15

D. 24

E. The answer cannot be determined from the information given

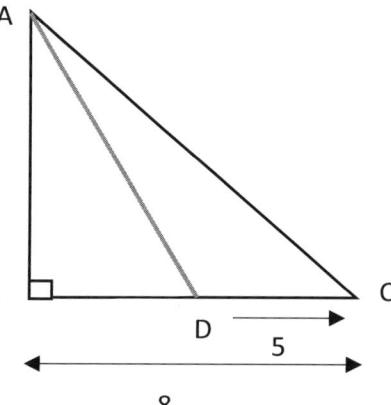

22) Which of the following is one solution of this equation?

$$x^2 + 2x - 5 = 0$$

A. $\sqrt{6} - 1$

B. $\sqrt{2} + 1$

C. $\sqrt{6} + 1$

D. $\sqrt{2} - 1$

E. $\sqrt{12}$

23) Two-kilograms apple and three-kilograms orange cost $26.4. If one-kilogram apple costs $4.2 how much does one-kilogram orange cost?

A. $9

B. $6

C. $5.5

D. $5

E. $4

24) A card is drawn at random from a standard 52–card deck, what is the probability that the card is of Hearts? (The deck includes 13 of each suit clubs, diamonds, hearts, and spades)

A. $\frac{1}{3}$

B. $\frac{1}{4}$

C. $\frac{1}{6}$

D. $\frac{1}{52}$

E. $\frac{1}{104}$

25) Which of the following expressions is equal to $\sqrt{\frac{x^2}{2} + \frac{x^2}{16}}$?

A. x

B. $\frac{3x}{4}$

C. $x\sqrt{x}$

D. $\frac{x\sqrt{x}}{4}$

E. $4x$

26) A football team had $20,000 to spend on supplies. The team spent $14,000 on new balls. New sport shoes cost $120 each. Which of the following inequalities represent how many new shoes the team can purchase.

   A. $120x + 14{,}000 \leq 20{,}000$
   B. $120x + 14{,}000 \geq 20{,}000$
   C. $14{,}000x + 120 \leq 20{,}000$
   D. $14{,}000x + 12{,}0 \geq 20{,}000$
   E. $14{,}000x + 1200 \geq 20{,}000$

27) If $\sqrt{6x} = \sqrt{y}$, then $x =$

   A. $6y$
   B. $\sqrt{\dfrac{y}{6}}$
   C. $\sqrt{6y}$
   D. y^2
   E. $\dfrac{y}{6}$

28) The average weight of 18 girls in a class is 60 kg and the average weight of 32 boys in the same class is 62 kg. What is the average weight of all the 50 students in that class?

   A. 60
   B. 61.28
   C. 61.68
   D. 61.90
   E. 62.20

29) If $y = (-3x^3)^2$, which of the following expressions is equal to y?

   A. $-6x^5$

   B. $-6x^6$

   C. $6x^5$

   D. $9x^5$

   E. $9x^6$

30) What is the value of the expression $5(x - 2y) + (2 - x)^2$ when $x = 3$ and $= -2$?

   A. -4

   B. 20

   C. 36

   D. 50

   E. 80

31) Sophia purchased a sofa for $530.40. The sofa is regularly priced at $624. What was the percent discount Sophia received on the sofa?

   A. 12%

   B. 15%

   C. 20%

   D. 25%

   E. 40%

32) The average of five consecutive numbers is 38. What is the smallest number?

   A. 38
   B. 36
   C. 34
   D. 12
   E. 8

33) The surface area of a cylinder is $150\pi\ cm^2$. If its height is 10 cm, what is the radius of the cylinder?

   A. 13 cm
   B. 11 cm
   C. 15 cm
   D. 5 cm
   E. 7 cm

34) What is the slope of a line that is perpendicular to the line
$$4x - 2y = 12?$$

   A. -2
   B. $-\frac{1}{2}$
   C. 4
   D. 12
   E. 14

35) What is the difference in area between a 9 cm by 4 cm rectangle and a circle with diameter of 10 cm? ($\pi = 3$)

   A. 49
   B. 39
   C. 6
   D. 4
   E. 2

36) If $f(x)=2x^3+ 2$ and $(x) = \frac{1}{x}$, what is the value of $f(g(x))$?

   A. $\frac{1}{2x^3+2}$
   B. $\frac{2}{x^3}$
   C. $\frac{1}{2x}$
   D. $\frac{1}{2x+2}$
   E. $\frac{2}{x^3} + 2$

37) A cruise line ship left Port A and traveled 80 miles due west and then 150 miles due north. At this point, what is the shortest distance from the cruise to port A?

   A. 70 miles
   B. 80 miles
   C. 150 miles
   D. 170 miles
   E. 230 miles

38) If the ratio of $5a$ to $2b$ is $\frac{1}{10}$, what is the ratio of a to b?

- A. 10
- B. 25
- C. $\frac{1}{25}$
- D. $\frac{1}{20}$
- E. $\frac{1}{10}$

39) If $x = 9$, what is the value of y in the following equation?

$$2y = \frac{2x^2}{3} + 6$$

- A. 30
- B. 45
- C. 60
- D. 120
- E. 180

40) The ratio of boys to girls in a school is 2:3. If there are 600 students in a school, how many boys are in the school.

- A. 540
- B. 360
- C. 300
- D. 280
- E. 240

The End of Practice Test 2

DAT Quantitative Reasoning Practice Tests Answers and Explanations

✳ Now, it's time to review your results to see where you went wrong and what areas you need to improve!

DAT Quantitative Reasoning Practice Tests Answer Key

DAT Practice Test 1

#	Ans	#	Ans	#	Ans
1	B	17	D	33	B
2	B	18	A	34	B
3	C	19	C	35	A
4	B	20	C	36	C
5	B	21	D	37	A
6	B	22	B	38	B
7	E	23	E	39	C
8	C	24	E	40	C
9	D	25	C		
10	C	26	B		
11	C	27	C		
12	B	28	D		
13	D	29	C		
14	B	30	E		
15	D	31	D		
16	C	32	E		

DAT Practice Test 2

#	Ans	#	Ans	#	Ans
1	A	17	D	33	D
2	A	18	C	34	B
3	B	19	A	35	B
4	E	20	A	36	E
5	E	21	D	37	D
6	C	22	A	38	C
7	C	23	B	39	A
8	E	24	B	40	E
9	A	25	B		
10	A	26	A		
11	C	27	E		
12	A	28	B		
13	D	29	E		
14	A	30	C		
15	B	31	B		
16	E	32	B		

DAT Quantitative Reasoning Practice Tests

Answers and Explanations

DAT Quantitative Reasoning Practice Test 1

1) **Choice B is correct**

To find the discount, multiply the number by (100% − rate of discount).

Therefore, for the first discount we get: (D) (100% − 20%) = (D) (0.80) = 0.80 D

For increase of 10 %: (0.85 D) (100% + 10%) = (0.85 D) (1.10) = 0.88 D = 88% of D

2) **Choice B is correct.**

1000 times the number is 40.5. Let x be the number, then:

$$1000x = 40.5$$

$$x = \frac{40.5}{1000} = 0.0405$$

3) **Choice C is correct**

The area of the floor is: 6 cm × 24 cm = 144 cm

The number is tiles needed = $144 \div 8 = 18$

4) Choice B is correct

The diagonal of the square is 8. Let x be the side.

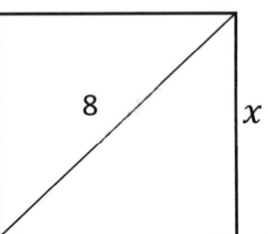

Use Pythagorean Theorem: $a^2 + b^2 = c^2$

$x^2 + x^2 = 8^2 \Rightarrow 2x^2 = 8^2 \Rightarrow 2x^2 = 64 \Rightarrow x^2 = 32 \Rightarrow x = \sqrt{32}$

The area of the square is:

$\sqrt{32} \times \sqrt{32} = 32$

5) Choice B is correct

$x = 20 + 125 = 145$

6) Choice B is correct.

By definition, the sine of any acute angle is equal to the cosine of its complement.

Since, angle A and B are complementary angles, therefore:

$$\sin A = \cos B$$

7) Choice E is correct

Solve the system of equations by elimination method.

$\begin{array}{l} 3x - 4y = -20 \\ -x + 2y = 10 \end{array}$ Multiply the second equation by 3, then add it to the first equation.

$\begin{array}{l} 3x - 4y = -20 \\ 3(-x + 2y = 10) \end{array} \Rightarrow \begin{array}{l} 3x - 4y = -20 \\ -3x + 6y = 30 \end{array} \Rightarrow$ add the equations

$2y = 10 \Rightarrow y = 5$

8) Choice C is correct

Use distance formula:

Distance = Rate × time ⇒ 420 = 50 × T, divide both sides by 50. 420 / 50 = T ⇒ T = 8.4 hours.

Change hours to minutes for the decimal part. 0.4 hours = 0.4 × 60 = 24 minutes.

9) Choice D is correct

x and z are colinear. y and $5x$ are colinear. Therefore,

$x + z = y + 5x$, subtract x from both sides, then, $z = y + 4x$

10) Choice C is correct

40% of 60 equals to: $0.40 \times 60 = 24$

12% of 600 equals to: $0.12 \times 600 = 72$

40% of 60 is added to 12% of 600: $24 + 72 = 96$

11) Choice C is correct

4% of the volume of the solution is alcohol. Let x be the volume of the solution.

Then: $4\%\ of\ x = 24\ ml \Rightarrow 0.04\ x = 24 \Rightarrow x = 24 \div 0.04 = 600$

12) Choice B is correct

Plug in each pair of number in the equation:

    A. $(2, 1)$: $2(2) + 4(1) = 8$ Nope!

    B. $(-1, 3)$: $2(-1) + 4(3) = 10$ Bingo!

    C. $(-2, 2)$: $2(-2) + 4(2) = 4$ Nope!

    D. $(2, 2)$: $2(2) + 4(2) = 12$ Nope!

    E. $(2, 8)$: $2(2) + 4(8) = 36$ Nope!

13) Choice D is correct

The area of ΔBED is 16, then: $\frac{4 \times AB}{2} = 16 \rightarrow 4 \times AB = 32 \rightarrow AB = 8$

The area of ΔBDF is 18, then: $\frac{3 \times BC}{2} = 18 \rightarrow 3 \times BC = 36 \rightarrow BC = 12$

The perimeter of the rectangle is $= 2 \times (8 + 12) = 40$

14) Choice B is correct

$|x - 10| \leq 3 \rightarrow -3 \leq x - 10 \leq 3 \rightarrow -3 + 10 \leq x - 10 + 10 \leq 3 + 10 \rightarrow 7 \leq x \leq 13$

15) Choice D is correct

If 17 balls are removed from the bag at random, there will be one ball in the bag. The probability of choosing a brown ball is 1 out of 18. Therefore, the probability of not choosing a brown ball is 17 out of 18 and the probability of having not a brown ball after removing 17 balls is the same.

16) Choice C is correct

Write a proportion and solve for x.

$\frac{3}{2} = \frac{x}{24} \Rightarrow 2x = 3 \times 24 \Rightarrow x = 36$ ft

17) Choice D is correct

The relationship among all sides of special right triangle

$30° - 60° - 90°$ is provided in this triangle:

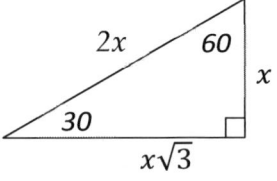

In this triangle, the opposite side of $30°$ angle is half of the hypotenuse.

Draw the shape of this question:

The latter is the hypotenuse. Therefore, the latter is 60 ft.

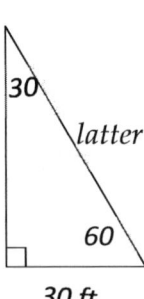

18) Choice A is correct

The percent of girls playing tennis is: $40\% \times 25\% = 0.40 \times 0.25 = 0.10 = 10\%$

19) Choice C is correct

Add the first 5 numbers. $40 + 45 + 50 + 35 + 55 = 225$

To find the distance traveled in the next 5 hours, multiply the average by number of hours.

$Distance = Average \times Rate = 50 \times 5 = 250$

Add both numbers. $250 + 225 = 475$

20) Choice C is correct

The question is this: 1.75 is what percent of 1.25?

Use percent formula:

$part = \frac{percent}{100} \times whole$

$1.75 = \frac{percent}{100} \times 1.25 \Rightarrow 1.75 = \frac{percent \times 1.25}{100} \Rightarrow 175 = percent \times 1.25 \Rightarrow percent = \frac{175}{1.25} = 140$

21) Choice D is correct.

Solve for x.

$\frac{3x}{16} = \frac{x-1}{4}$

Multiply the second fraction by 4.

$\frac{3x}{16} = \frac{4(x-1)}{4 \times 4}$

Tow denominators are equal. Therefore, the numerators must be equal.

$3x = 4x - 4$

$0 = x - 4$

$4 = x$

22) Choice B is correct

$$tan\theta = \frac{opposite}{adjacent}$$

$tan\theta = \frac{5}{12} \Rightarrow$ we have the following right triangle. Then

$c = \sqrt{5^2 + 12^2} = \sqrt{25 + 144} = \sqrt{169} = 13$

$cos\theta = \frac{adjacent}{hypotenuse} = \frac{12}{13}$

23) Choice E is correct

$0.6x = (0.3) \times 20 \rightarrow x = 10 \rightarrow (x + 5)^2 = (15)^2 = 225$

24) Choice E is correct

The slop of line A is: $m = \frac{y_2 - y_1}{x_2 - x_1} = \frac{3-2}{4-3} = 1$

Parallel lines have the same slope and only choice E (y = x) has slope of 1.

25) Choice C is correct

When points are reflected over y-axis, the value of y in the coordinates doesn't change and the sign of x changes. Therefore, the coordinates of point B is $(-10, 3)$.

26) Choice B is correct

The area of trapezoid is: $\left(\frac{8+12}{2}\right) \times x = 100 \rightarrow 10x = 100 \rightarrow x = 10$

$$y = \sqrt{3^2 + 4^2} = 5$$

Perimeter is: $12 + 10 + 8 + 5 = 35$

27) Choice C is correct

Set of number that are not composite between 1 and 25: $A = \{1, 2, 3, 5, 7, 11, 13, 17, 19, 23\}$

$$\text{Probability} = \frac{\text{number of desired outcomes}}{\text{number of total outcomes}} = \frac{10}{25} = \frac{2}{5}$$

28) Choice D is correct

Check each option provided:

A. 1 $\dfrac{4+5+8+11+\ }{5} = \dfrac{40}{5} = 8$

B. 4 $\dfrac{1+5+8+11+12}{5} = \dfrac{37}{5} = 7.4$

C. 5 $\dfrac{1+4+8+11+\ }{5} = \dfrac{36}{5} = 7.2$

D. 11 $\dfrac{1+4+5+8+12}{5} = \dfrac{30}{5} = 6$

E. 12 $\dfrac{1+4+5+8+11}{5} = \dfrac{29}{5} = 5.8$

29) Choice C is correct

The weight of 12.2 meters of this rope is: $12.2 \times 600\ g = 7320\ g$

$1\ kg = 1000\ g$, therefore, $7320\ g \div 1000 = 7.32\ kg$

30) Choice E is correct

$y = 4ab + 3b^3 +$

Plug in the values of a and b in the equation: $a = 2$ and $b = 3$

$y = 4(2)(3) + 3(3)^3 = 24 + 3(27) = 24 + 81 = 105$

31) Choice D is correct

$(g - f)(x) = g(x) - f(x) = (-x^2 - 1 - 2x) - (5 + x)$

$-x^2 - 1 - 2x - 5 - x = -x^2 - 3x - 6$

32) Choice E is correct

$g(x) = -2$, then $f(g(x)) = f(-2) = 2(-2)^3 + 5(-2)^2 + 2(-2) = -16 + 20 - 4 = 0$

33) Choice B is correct

Plug in $z/3$ for z and simplify.

$$x_1 = \frac{8y + \frac{r}{r+1}}{\frac{6}{\frac{z}{3}}} = \frac{8y + \frac{r}{r+1}}{\frac{3 \times 6}{z}} = \frac{8y + \frac{r}{r+1}}{3 \times \frac{6}{z}} = \frac{1}{3} \times \frac{8y + \frac{r}{r+1}}{\frac{6}{z}} = \frac{x}{3}$$

34) Choice B is correct

Use the information provided in the question to draw the shape.

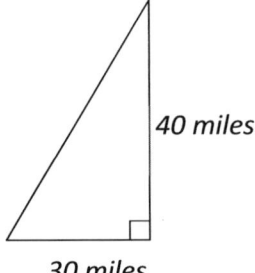

Use Pythagorean Theorem: $a^2 + b^2 = c^2$

$40^2 + 30^2 = c^2 \Rightarrow 1600 + 900 = c^2 \Rightarrow 2500 = c^2 \Rightarrow c = 50$

35) Choice A is correct.

Let the number be A. Then: $x = y\% \times A$

Solve for A. $x = \frac{y}{100} \times A$

Multiply both sides by $\frac{100}{y}$:

$$x \times \frac{100}{y} = \frac{y}{100} \times \frac{100}{y} \times A$$

$$A = \frac{100x}{y}$$

36) Choice C is correct

$$tangent\ \beta = \frac{1}{cotangent\ \beta} = \frac{1}{1} = 1$$

37) Choice A is correct

One liter = 1000 cm³ → 6 liters = 6000 cm³

$6000 = 15 \times 5 \times h \rightarrow h = \frac{6000}{75} = 80$ cm

38) Choice B is correct

$\frac{2}{3} \times 90 = 60$

39) Choice C is correct

I. $|a| < 1 \to -1 < a < 1$

Multiply all sides by b. Since, $b > 0 \to -b < ba < b$ (it is true!)

II. Since, $-1 < a < 1, and\ a < 0 \to -a > a^2 > a$ (plug in $-\frac{1}{2}$, and check!) (It's false)

III. $-1 < a < 1, multiply\ all\ sides\ by\ 2, then: -2 < 2a < 2$

Subtract 3 from all sides. Then:

$-2 - 3 < 2a - 3 < 2 - 3 \to -5 < 2a - 3 < -1$ (It is true!)

40) Choice C is correct

Surface Area of a cylinder = $2\pi r\ (r + h)$,

The radius of the cylinder is $3(6 \div 2)$ inches and its height is 8 inches. Therefore,

Surface Area of a cylinder $= 2\pi(3)(3 + 8) = 66\pi$

DAT Quantitative Reasoning Practice Test 2

1) **Choice A is correct**

$$\left(\frac{f}{g}\right)(x) = \frac{f(x)}{g(x)} = \frac{3x-1}{x^2-x}$$

2) **Choice A is correct.**

The equation of a line is: $y = mx + b$, where m is the slope and b is the y-intercept.

First find the slope:

$$m = \frac{y_2 - y_1}{x_2 - x_1} = \frac{15 - (-5)}{8 - 3} = \frac{20}{5} = 4$$

Then, we have: $y = 4x + b$

Choose one point and plug in the values of x and y in the equation to solve for b.

Let's choose the point $(3, -5)$

$$y = 4x + b \to -5 = 4(3) + b \to -5 = 12 + b \to b = -17$$

The equation of the line is: $y = 4x - 17$

3) **Choice B is correct**

Use simple interest formula:

$I = prt$

(I = interest, p = principal, r = rate, t = time)

$$I = (12000)(0.035)(2) = 840$$

4) **Choice E is correct**

Number of visiting fans: $\frac{2 \times 25000}{5} = 10,000$

5) **Choice E is correct.**

The sum of all angles in a quadrilateral is 360 degrees.

Let x be the smallest angle in the quadrilateral. Then the angles are:

$$x, 2x, 2x, 5x$$

$$x + 2x + 2x + 5x = 360 \rightarrow 10x = 360 \rightarrow x = 36$$

The angles in the quadrilateral are: 36°, 72°, 72°, and 180°

6) **Choice C is correct.**

Formula for the area of a circle is:

$$A = \pi r^2$$

Using 64 for the area of the circle we have:

$$64 = \pi r^2$$

Let's solve for the radius (r).

$$\frac{64}{\pi} = r^2 \rightarrow r = \sqrt{\frac{64}{\pi}} = \frac{8}{\sqrt{\pi}} = \frac{8}{\sqrt{\pi}} \times \frac{\sqrt{\pi}}{\sqrt{\pi}} = \frac{8\sqrt{\pi}}{\pi}$$

7) **Choice C is correct**

Length of the rectangle is: $\frac{5}{4} \times 16 = 20$

perimeter of rectangle is: $2 \times (20 + 16) = 72$

8) **Choice E is correct**

The angle x and 35 are complementary angles. Therefore:

$$x + 35 = 180$$

$180° - 35° = 145°$

9) Choice A is correct

Three times of 24,000 is 72,000. One sixth of them cancelled their tickets.

One sixth of 72,000 equals 12,000 ($\frac{1}{6} \times 72000 = 12000$).

60,000 (72000 − 12000 = 60000) fans are attending this week

10) Choice A is correct

$sinA = \frac{1}{3} \Rightarrow$

Since $sin\theta = \frac{opposite}{hypotenus}$, we have the following right triangle. Then:

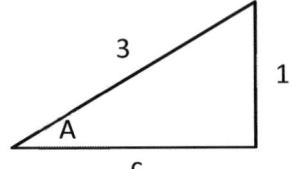

$c = \sqrt{3^2 - 1^2} = \sqrt{9 - 1} = \sqrt{8}$

$cosA = \frac{\sqrt{8}}{3}$

11) Choice C is correct

Plug in the value of each option in the inequality.

A. 1 $(1 − 2)^2 + 1 > 3(1) − 1 \rightarrow 2 > 2$ No!

B. 6 $(6 − 2)^2 + 1 > 3(6) − 1 \rightarrow 17 > 17$ No!

C. 8 $(8 − 2)^2 + 1 > 3(8) − 1 \rightarrow 37 > 23$ Bingo!

D. 3 $(3 − 2)^2 + 1 > 3(3) − 1 \rightarrow 2 > 8$ No!

E. 4 $(4 − 2)^2 + 1 > 3(4) − 1 \rightarrow 5 > 11$ No!

12) Choice A is correct

First, find the number.

Let x be the number. Write the equation and solve for x.

150 % of a number is 75, then:

$1.5 \times x = 75 \Rightarrow x = 75 \div 1.5 = 50$

90 % of 50 is:

$0.9 \times 50 = 45$

13) Choice D is correct

If the length of the box is 27, then the width of the box is one third of it, 9, and the height of the box is 3 (one third of the width). The volume of the box is:

$V = (length) \times (width) \times (height) = (27) \times (9) \times (3) = 729$

14) Choice A is correct

$x - 2 \geq 3 \rightarrow x \geq 3 + 2 \rightarrow x \geq 5$

Or

$x - 2 \leq -3 \rightarrow x \leq -3 + 2 \rightarrow x \leq -1$

Then, solution is: $\quad x \geq 5 \cup x \leq -1$

15) Choice B is correct.

$\tan = \frac{opposite}{adjacent}$, and $\tan x = \frac{8}{15}$, therefore, the opposite side of the angle x is 8 and the adjacent side is 15. Let's draw the triangle.

Using Pythagorean theorem, we have:

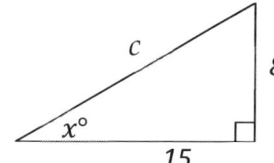

$a^2 + b^2 = c^2 \rightarrow 8^2 + 15^2 = c^2 \rightarrow 64 + 225 = c^2 \rightarrow c = 17$

$$\sin x = \frac{opposite}{hypotenuse} = \frac{8}{17}$$

16) Choice E is correct

Based on triangle similarity theorem: $\frac{a}{a+b} = \frac{c}{3} \rightarrow c = \frac{3a}{a+b} = \frac{3\sqrt{3}}{3\sqrt{3}} = 1 \rightarrow$ area of shaded region is:

$\left(\frac{c+3}{2}\right)(b) = \frac{4}{2} \times 2\sqrt{3} = 4\sqrt{3}$

17) Choice D is correct

$670000 = 6.7 \times 10^5$

18) Choice C is correct

the population is increased by 15% and 20%. 15% increase changes the population to 115% of original population.

For the second increase, multiply the result by 120%.

$(1.15) \times (1.20) = 1.38 = 138\%$

38 percent of the population is increased after two years.

19) Choice A is correct

$(x^6)^{\frac{5}{8}} = x^{6 \times \frac{5}{8}} = x^{\frac{30}{8}} = x^{\frac{15}{4}}$

20) Choice A is correct.

The relationship among all sides of right triangle $30° - 60° - 90°$ is provided in the following triangle:

Sine of 30° equals to: $\frac{opposite}{hypotenuse} = \frac{x}{2x} = \frac{1}{2}$

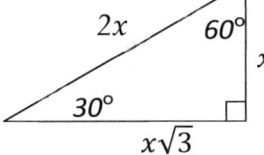

21) Choice D is correct

Let x be the length of AB, then:

$$15 = \frac{x \times 5}{2} \rightarrow x = 6$$

The length of AC $= \sqrt{6^2 + 8^2} = \sqrt{100} = 10$

The perimeter of $\triangle ABC = 6 + 8 + 10 = 24$

22) Choice A is correct

$$x_{1,2} = \frac{-b \pm \sqrt{b^2 - 4ac}}{2a}$$

$ax^2 + bx + c = 0$

$x^2 + 2x - 5 = 0 \quad \Rightarrow \quad$ then: $a = 1, b = 2$ and $c = -5$

$$x = \frac{-2 + \sqrt{2^2 - 4.1.-5}}{2.1} = \sqrt{6} - 1 \qquad x = \frac{-2 - \sqrt{2^2 - 4.1.-5}}{2.1} = -1 - \sqrt{6}$$

23) Choice B is correct

Let x be the cost of one-kilogram orange, then: $\quad 3x + (2 \times 4.2) = 26.4 \rightarrow$

$$3x + 8.4 = 26.4 \rightarrow 3x = 26.4 - 8.4 \rightarrow 3x = 18 \rightarrow x = \frac{18}{3} = \$6$$

24) Choice B is correct

The probability of choosing a Hearts is $\frac{13}{52} = \frac{1}{4}$

25) Choice B is correct.

Simplify the expression.

$$\sqrt{\frac{x^2}{2} + \frac{x^2}{16}} = \sqrt{\frac{8x^2}{16} + \frac{x^2}{16}} = \sqrt{\frac{9x^2}{16}} = \sqrt{\frac{9}{16}x^2} =$$

$$\sqrt{\frac{9}{16}} \times \sqrt{x^2} = \frac{3}{4} \times x = \frac{3x}{4}$$

26) Choice A is correct

Let x be the number of shoes the team can purchase. Therefore, the team can purchase $120\ x$.

The team had $20,000 and spent $14000. Now the team can spend on new shoes $6000 at most.

Now, write the inequality:

$120x + 14,000 \leq 20,000$

27) Choice E is correct.

Solve for x.

$$\sqrt{6x} = \sqrt{y}$$

Square both sides of the equation:

$$(\sqrt{6x})^2 = (\sqrt{y})^2$$

$$6x = y$$

$$x = \frac{y}{6}$$

28) Choice B is correct

$$\text{average} = \frac{\text{sum of terms}}{\text{number of terms}}$$

The sum of the weight of all girls is: $18 \times 60 = 1080\ kg$

The sum of the weight of all boys is: $32 \times 62 = 1984\ kg$

The sum of the weight of all students is: $1080 + 1984 = 3064\ kg$

$$\text{average} = \frac{3064}{50} = 61.28$$

29) Choice E is correct.

$$y = (-3x^3)^2 = (-3)^2(x^3)^2 = 9x^6$$

30) Choice C is correct

Plug in the value of x and y.

$x = 3$ and $y = -2$

$5(x-2y)+(2-x)^2 = 5(3-2(-2))+(2-3)^2 = 5(3+4)+(-1)^2 = 35+1 = 36$

31) Choice B is correct

The question is this: 530.40 is what percent of 624?

Use percent formula:

$$\text{part} = \frac{\text{percent}}{100} \times \text{whole}$$

$530.40 = \frac{\text{percent}}{100} \times 624 \Rightarrow 530.40 = \frac{\text{percent} \times 624}{100} \Rightarrow 53040 = \text{percent} \times 624 \Rightarrow$

$\text{percent} = \frac{53040}{624} = 85$

530.40 is 85 % of 624. Therefore, the discount is: 100% − 85% = 15%

32) Choice B is correct

Let x be the smallest number. Then, these are the numbers:

$x, x+1, x+2, x+3, x+4$

$\text{average} = \frac{\text{sum of terms}}{\text{number of terms}} \Rightarrow 38 = \frac{x+(x+1)+(x+2)+(x+3)+(x+4)}{5} \Rightarrow 38 = \frac{5x+10}{5} \Rightarrow 190 = 5x+10 \Rightarrow$

$180 = 5x \Rightarrow x = 36$

33) Choice D is correct

Formula for the Surface area of a cylinder is:
$$SA = 2\pi r^2 + 2\pi rh \rightarrow 150\pi = 2\pi r^2 + 2\pi r(10) \rightarrow r^2 + 10r - 75 = 0$$
Factorize and solve for r.

$$(r+15)(r-5) = 0 \rightarrow r = 5 \quad \text{or} \quad r = -15 \ (unacceptable)$$

34) Choice B is correct

The equation of a line in slope intercept form is: $y = mx + b$

Solve for y.

$4x - 2y = 12 \Rightarrow -2y = 12 - 4x \Rightarrow y = (12 - 4x) \div (-2) \Rightarrow$

$y = 2x - 6$

The slope is 2.

The slope of the line perpendicular to this line is:

$m_1 \times m_2 = -1 \Rightarrow 2 \times m_2 = -1 \Rightarrow m_2 = -\frac{1}{2}$

35) Choice B is correct

The area of rectangle is: $9 \times 4 = 36$ cm²

The area of circle is: $\pi r^2 = \pi \times (\frac{10}{2})^2 = 3 \times 25 = 75$ cm²

Difference of areas is: $75 - 36 = 39$

36) Choice E is correct

$f(g(x)) = 2 \times (\frac{1}{x})^3 + 2 = \frac{2}{x^3} + 2$

37) Choice D is correct

Use the information provided in the question to draw the shape.

Use Pythagorean Theorem: $a^2 + b^2 = c^2$

$80^2 + 150^2 = c^2 \Rightarrow 6400 + 22500 = c^2 \Rightarrow 28900 = c^2 \Rightarrow c = 170$

38) Choice C is correct

Write the ratio of $5a$ to $2b$. $\frac{5a}{2b} = \frac{1}{10}$

Use cross multiplication and then simplify. $5a \times 10 = 2b \times 1 \rightarrow 50a = 2b \rightarrow a = \frac{2b}{50} = \frac{b}{25}$

Now, find the ratio of a to b. $\frac{a}{b} = \frac{\frac{b}{25}}{b} \rightarrow \frac{b}{25} \div b = \frac{b}{25} \times \frac{1}{b} = \frac{b}{25b} = \frac{1}{25}$

39) Choice A is correct

Plug in the value of x in the equation and solve for y.

$$2y = \frac{2x^2}{3} + 6 \rightarrow 2y = \frac{2(9)^2}{3} + 6 \rightarrow 2y = \frac{2(81)}{3} + 6 \rightarrow 2y = 54 + 6 = 60$$

$$2y = 60 \rightarrow y = 30$$

40) Choice E is correct

The ratio of boy to girls is 2:3. Therefore, there are 2 boys out of 5 students. To find the answer, first divide the total number of students by 5, then multiply the result by 2.

$600 \div 5 = 120 \Rightarrow 120 \times 2 = 240$

www.EffortlessMath.com

... So Much More Online!

✓ FREE Math lessons

✓ More Math learning books!

✓ Mathematics Worksheets

✓ Online Math Tutors

Need a PDF version of this book?

Please visit www.EffortlessMath.com